Concussion: What has happened to my brain?

A practical guide to recovery

Dr Peter O. Jenkins, BMBCh, MA, PhD

Copyright © 2021 Peter Jenkins All rights reserved

The characters and events portrayed in this book are fictitious. Any similarity to real persons, living or dead, is coincidental and not intended by the author.

No part of this book may be reproduced, or stored in a retrieval system, or transmitted in any form or by any means, electronic, mechanical, photocopying, recording, or otherwise, without express written permission of the publisher.

ISBN-13: 9798700787956

Contents

INTRODUCTION 1

PART 1: WHAT IS CONCUSSION? 9

    What is concussion? 11
    What happens to the brain during and after trauma? 21
    Why do some people have persistent symptoms? 29
    What are the long-term consequences? 37
    How can I get better? 45

PART 2: SYMPTOMS AFTER A CONCUSSION 53

    1. Headache 55
    2. Anxiety and low mood/depression 67
    3. Post-traumatic stress symptoms 73
    4. Difficulties with memory, concentration and speed of thinking 81
    5. Dizziness and feeling unsteady 93
    6. Light and sound sensitivity 107
    7. Sleep disturbance and fatigue 109
    8. Irritability and other changes in personality 119
    9. Problems with vision 121
    10. Hearing problems 125

PART 3: SPECIFIC ISSUES FOLLOWING A CONCUSSION 131

    Getting back to work, exercise and education 133
    Return to contact sports 139
    Diet and supplements 145
    "Brain-Training" 149
    Driving and flying 153

WHERE TO GET EXTRA HELP 157

Acknowledgements:

I would like to thank Harriet Jones for her amazing design skills, Paul Jenkins for his editorial input, my parents, and especially P, F, J and M for their support, love and encouragement.

Introduction

"Concussions" are common. It is estimated that half of us will suffer one at some point in our life.

But what is a "concussion", what has happened to the brain and is it permanent?

These are important and frequently asked questions, yet surprisingly we do not have good answers to them. For example, there is no single, universally accepted definition for what constitutes a concussion. This may seem odd, especially as it is such a commonly used term, but it is used in a variety of ways referring to different things. Sometimes it is used to describe the minor head injury itself, sometimes to describe the symptoms experienced *after* a head injury (e.g. headache, dizziness and concentration problems) and sometimes to describe the physical injury that has happened to the brain (i.e. my brain is concussed).

Does this matter? Is an agreed definition for concussion that important? You might say that most of us understand what we mean by the term concussion and that the lack of a precise definition is unimportant for its everyday use. However, in my experience, I find that the differing interpretations of the word can lead to confusion and misunderstanding, which in turn can lead to a prolongation of symptoms after a head injury. For these reasons, and because the term "concussion" is here to stay, I think it is a useful start to consider potential issues that can arise from variable usage of the term.

Often, my impression is that people prefer to use the term concussion because the alternative, i.e. a brain injury, can seem very scary. The mention of brain injury can conjure up images of some awful long-lasting damage to our brains. This is rarely the case following a minor head injury, even in the situation when symptoms persist. I will discuss how the brain is affected by a head injury and why ongoing symptoms may not necessarily be due to permanent damage to the brain. In fact, in the case of a minor head injury, persistent symptoms are *rarely* due to structural injury to the brain.

People with prolonged symptoms after a concussion are frequently told:

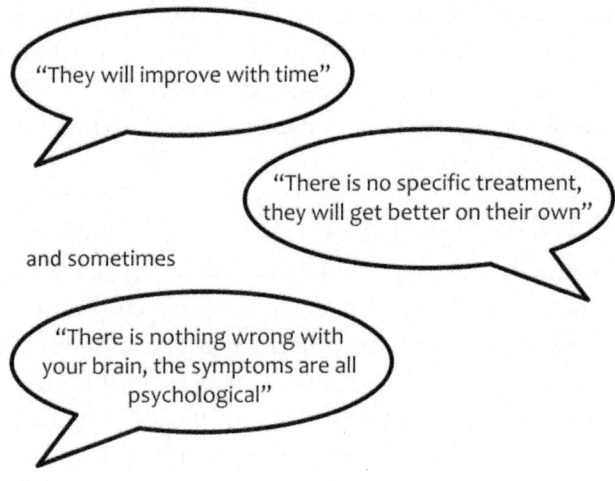

Around 1 in 5 people will have symptoms lasting beyond 3 months after a mild head injury. For those suffering persistent symptoms it can feel like you are the only person in the world with these problems. This is because the symptoms suffered are often invisible to those around you, for example headaches, dizziness, low mood, anxiety, and memory problems. This is why it has become known as the "hidden disability" with symptoms often being under-recognised and frequently under-treated.

I will explore the reasons for persistent symptoms and discuss how they can (and often should) be treated. Time may be the greatest healer, but this is not always the case for persistent symptoms after a minor head injury when recognition of the cause and appropriate treatment is often necessary. It is also important to recognise the link between physical and psychological factors and that the two often intertwine. It is too simplistic to divide causes between the purely physical and the entirely psychological. This approach is unhelpful as the two factors often co-exist with the first commonly driving the second (or vice-versa): who would not feel down and depressed if they were suffering chronic pain?

Beyond the risk of the immediate problems caused by a head injury there is also a growing recognition that, in some people, minor repeated head injuries can cause problems many years after the event. It has become well-publicised that repeated minor head injuries are associated with an increased risk of dementia. This is obviously an area of major concern, particularly within the context of sporting injuries where minor head injuries are frequently encountered, even in sports that are considered non-contact. There has been a great deal of confusion regarding what is meant by dementia in this situation. Most of us relate the term dementia to a disease where memory and other brain functions decline over time more rapidly than we would expect with normal ageing. Alzheimer's disease is the common example that many of us will have unfortunately encountered in others. In the context of repeated, minor head injuries a disease process called chronic traumatic encephalopathy, also referred to as CTE and previously known as punch-drunk syndrome or dementia pugilistica, has been described. CTE is a disease that, like Alzheimer's disease, appears to cause an accelerated and progressive loss of brain cells and thereby brain function over time. It is important, however, to realise that there is much we do not know about this condition and much more research is needed to define how common it is and who might be at risk.

In addition to describing a process of progressive decline in brain function such as that seen in CTE and Alzheimer's disease, dementia can also be used to describe a 'fixed' or 'static' impairment in brain function. In other words, the brain may not be working as well in processes such as memory and thinking as before but it is **not** worsening over time. It is therefore important to disentangle impairments in brain function that are related to a progressive disease process and those that are static and not worsening as this has clear implications for the future.

Finally, on the issue of dementia, it is important to remember that there are many reasons why the brain may not be working as well as it should. Pain, depression, anxiety, post-traumatic stress symptoms, impaired sleep and balance issues will all impair our other brain processes including memory and concentration. Therefore, before concluding that symptoms are due to dementia, it is important to make sure these other factors are looked for and addressed. I will discuss some of these issues and the current scientific understanding regarding the risks surrounding dementia after minor head injuries.

Reassuringly, there is a growing understanding in both the medical and public worlds of the significant problems that a concussion or mild brain injury can cause. If you are suffering from ongoing issues do not be afraid to seek medical advice as you will often be surprised how much can be done to help you. Moreover, it is important to stress that, from experiences of treating people who have suffered a brain injury, it is clear that a great number of problems can often be resolved – or at least improved – if the person understands the nature of their problem. For example, people are often surprised how long it can take symptoms to resolve. Unrealistic expectations as to how quickly symptoms will resolve can lead to anxiety. This will often prolong the symptoms and a vicious cycle may ensue.

Another common problem I encounter is the misunderstanding of the basis of someone's problems. For example, even minor head injuries can trigger migraines. Migraines produce a constellation of symptoms including dizziness, sleep problems and difficulty concentrating. All these symptoms may be, understandably, attributed to the head injury, whereas, by treating the migraines, the secondary symptoms will also frequently resolve.

The purpose of this book is to empower an individual who has suffered a concussion by providing information about what has happened to the brain and the basis of the common problems experienced. It is true that most people will get completely back to normal after a concussion as most symptoms are self-limiting. It is therefore helpful to remain optimistic and to realise that sometimes it takes longer than expected to feel completely back to normal.

For the minority of people in whom symptoms persist, recovery can be aided by both an understanding of what has happened to the brain following an injury and how to treat specific symptoms. This book aims to provide an understanding of what has happened to the brain and the possible causes of lasting symptoms, but it does not replace a comprehensive assessment by a healthcare team trained in the management of head injuries as their help may be needed to treat certain symptoms.

In summary, the aims of this book are to explain what "concussion" is, the common symptoms experienced because of it, how these symptoms can be treated and, vitally, to de-bunk some of the common myths surrounding concussion.

How to use this book

The initial chapters discuss what concussion is, some of the common pitfalls that can lead to under-treatment and what is happening to the brain during and after a minor head injury. These chapters provide quite detailed information that some readers may want to skip but they do explain our current understanding and what we do not yet know. Later in the book, I discuss a general approach to self-management of symptoms after a minor head injury and then go into detailed management of specific symptoms. The general principles will hopefully be useful to all readers and then specific symptoms can be chosen based on need.

PART 1:
What is concussion?

What is concussion?

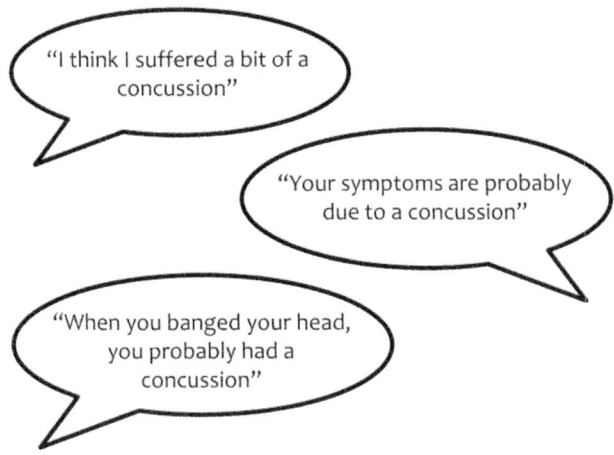

These are all common phrases that we hear. Concussion is a word that is familiar to nearly all of us and is frequently used by the media, especially in the context of the latest sporting star who has suffered a head injury. We also hear it used by medical professionals and may even have been diagnosed with it in the past by our doctor, but what does concussion mean exactly?

Surprisingly, there is no clear agreement on the definition of concussion. Sometimes it is used to describe the bang on the head itself: "I think you had a concussion", other times it is used to describe the symptoms experienced afterwards: "I think you're suffering from a concussion", and sometimes people use it to describe the injury to their brain: "my brain is concussed".

Most people use concussion to describe a blow (or jolting) to the head that causes symptoms, commonly headache, dizziness, and impaired concentration. It is therefore generally considered to be a *type* of traumatic brain injury but, rather than resulting in permanent injury to the brain it is often viewed as a transient, self-limiting phenomenon with no persistent brain damage.

> **Common symptoms after a head injury**
>
> Headache
> Dizziness
> Nausea and/or vomiting
> Poor concentration
> Slowed speed of thinking
> Sensitivity to noise and/or light
> Sleep disturbance
> Fatigue
> Feeling depressed or down
> Anxiety
> Irritability
> Forgetfulness or poor memory
> Blurred vision

The roots of the concept of concussion date back over a thousand years when early doctors started to differentiate between traumatic injuries to the brain that led to *structural* damage and bleeding in and around the brain and those injuries that led to a *transient* disruption to normal brain function caused by a "shaking" of the brain.

This idea of a separation between structural injury and injury without structural changes but a change in brain function has remained in both the lay and medical worlds. However, this distinction is not clear-cut, and important overlaps exist between the two. At what level do we consider there to be evidence of a structural injury? Do we have to see bleeding and damage to the brain on simple inspection or a CT scan? What if the brain looks normal to the naked eye but under a microscope we can see damage to the brain cells and blood vessels? This artificial distinction has led to confusion as to exactly what differentiates a concussion from a traumatic brain injury. There is clearly a continuum in the severity of traumatic injuries to the brain, from the very mildest (such as banging your head on a cabinet door) to the most severe road traffic accident resulting in coma and brain cell death and injury. For this reason, most people now recognise concussion as a mild form of traumatic brain injury and concussion is often used interchangeably with the term "mild traumatic brain injury".

But do these issues around the definition of concussion matter? After all, most of us understand that it describes a bang to the head and the symptoms experienced afterwards. For the most part, the exact definition of the term concussion is not necessarily that important – it is a word that most of us can both relate to and understand what it means when we use it. However, differences in interpretation can prove problematic in certain situations and have the potential to misinform, prevent proper treatment and ultimately lead to someone suffering needlessly. It is worth being a little more careful with our definition because, in my view, imprecise use of the term concussion has two main risks that we need to be conscious of:

First, a concussion is assumed to be a transient phenomenon; in other words, after a blow to the head, you may suffer some symptoms but the presumption is that these are due to a *transient* disruption to normal brain function and will self-resolve with time. Therefore, the assumption is that nothing needs to, or indeed should be, done as time and rest will resolve all symptoms. However, we know that 1 in 5 people will suffer symptoms for more than 3 months even after a mild head injury. This raises the obvious question of how can we diagnose a concussion at the time of injury if resolution of symptoms is necessary for the diagnosis but cannot be known at this time? This implicit assumption that a concussion is a transient phenomenon also poses the risk of a lack of engagement by health care professionals as they assume nothing needs to be done.

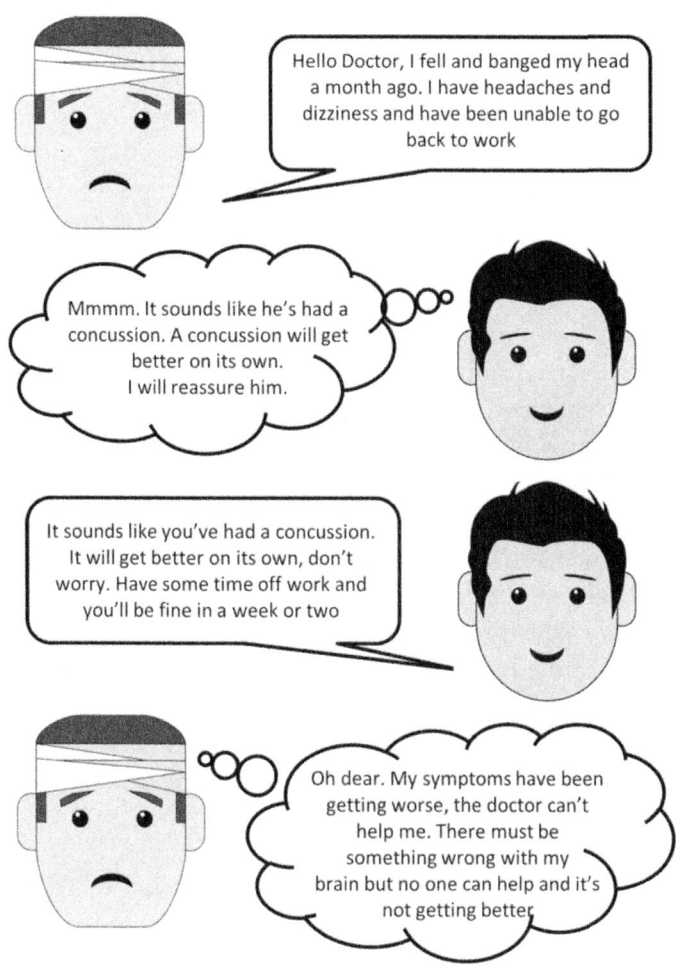

This incorrect assumption can lead to individuals' missing out on treatment that may improve their symptoms and people are often left confused as to why they still do not feel completely well despite being assured they should be back to normal. This confusion and concern may compound the existing symptoms. Although the doctor is usually not dismissing or not believing the symptoms, this is how it may come across to the patient who can feel alone and unsupported and be left with the assumption that nothing can be done to help them.

It is not uncommon for me to see a patient who has seen several health care professionals who have reassured them that their 'dizziness' or 'headache' will get better, but then things don't improve. Frequently, there is a treatable cause such as benign paroxysmal positional vertigo (see Dizziness section) or migraine. Compare this to the scenario where you see your doctor for a headache or dizziness but *without* a history of a head injury. In this situation, the doctor will take a history and examine you, diagnose the problem and advise a treatment. However, if the symptoms developed *after* a head injury, the assumption that they are transient and will resolve spontaneously can lead to a failure to properly assess and treat the complaint.

This brings us to the second reason why the term concussion and its connotations can hinder treatment. Concussion is sometimes used to refer to the *symptoms* suffered after a head injury, or more commonly people will refer to *post-concussion syndrome* to describe the constellation of symptoms suffered after a head injury. Therefore, someone presenting with persistent symptoms following a head injury is frequently diagnosed as having post-concussion syndrome. This is problematic for several reasons:

First, there are many different causes of persistent symptoms after a head injury, e.g. migraine, exacerbation of an underlying mental health disorder such as depression, post-traumatic stress disorder, and/or damage to the vestibular system (the balance apparatus in our inner ear). These causes all have different, specific treatments but if the underlying cause(s) for an individual's symptoms are not worked out and they are instead lumped together under the common label of "post-concussion syndrome", potentially helpful, specific treatments for certain symptoms may be ignored.

Second, it is presumed that injury to the brain after a concussion or mild head injury will resolve within three months. Therefore, anyone reporting symptoms beyond three months is presumed to have a 'psychological' cause for the persistence of symptoms. It is true that certain psychological factors can prolong symptoms, but it is not the case that **all** persistent symptoms are due to purely psychological factors. The important outcome of this is that psychological treatments cannot be expected to successfully treat all causes of persistent symptoms. For all these reasons, using a generic, non-specific term (such as concussion or post-concussion syndrome) to describe symptoms after a head injury carries the risk of limiting or even closing off the diagnostic process. This then prevents an accurate identification of why a particular individual has persistent symptoms and therefore misses the opportunity for appropriate treatment.

The concept that all persistent symptoms beyond three months are of a psychological nature has been compounded by the rise of litigation and medicolegal processes surrounding head injuries. Historically, there has been a belief that these processes have driven the persistence of symptoms after mild head injuries and persistent symptoms have even been called a "compensation neurosis". We shall discuss this more later and, in short, there is likely to be some element of truth in this assumption. However, by no means does it account for all persistent symptoms and **should not** be assumed to be the cause in an individual who is undergoing a medicolegal process.

What term should we use instead of concussion then?

We do not need to banish the term concussion to the scrap heap as it can be useful. It is a term that most of us can relate to and understand, but it is important to recognise the potential for confusion because of the issues discussed above.

To help prevent these biases it makes more sense to describe the nature and severity of the head injury suffered, e.g. a mild head injury caused by a fall with a brief period of feeling dazed but no loss of consciousness is very different to the severe traumatic brain injury caused by a high-speed car crash causing a prolonged coma and extensive bleeding in the brain. The former event is likely to result in full recovery with no residual symptoms whereas it would not be surprising if the latter resulted in multiple residual symptoms.

In the event of persisting symptoms, it is important to firstly identify the individual symptoms (e.g. headache, depression, dizziness etc.) and to then identify their specific causes by making specific diagnoses. For example, someone suffering headache, dizziness and irritability after a minor head injury may have developed or exacerbated migrainous headaches because migraine can be responsible for all these symptoms. Alternatively, someone reporting increased anxiety, fatigue, concentration difficulties and sleep disturbance may have exacerbated an underlying anxiety disorder. These two distinct diagnoses have very different treatment options. However, if, instead of this specific diagnostic approach, both individuals in the examples cited above were diagnosed with "post-concussion syndrome", the very different causes for their persistent symptoms would be missed and important treatment options may be denied as a result.

As we shall see, the severity of residual symptoms after head injury is not necessarily proportional to the extent of any underlying brain damage and it is important to separate these two aspects (i.e. the severity of brain injury and the resultant symptoms) to avoid assumptions that may risk inadequate treatment. By this I mean that a mild injury does not necessarily equate to no prolonged symptoms. In fact, we know that headaches are actually and, surprisingly, more common after a minor brain injury than after a severe one.

In the interests of clarity, I will generally refer to mild head injuries throughout the rest of this book rather than using the term concussion to avoid confusion between post-trauma symptoms and the injury itself.

What happens to the brain during and after trauma?

The brain is a relatively delicate structure and is enclosed within the hard, bony skull to protect it from injury. However, a sufficiently powerful blow to the head or a rapid acceleration/deceleration of the head (for example in a road traffic accident) will injure the brain. The skull is very good at protecting the brain from direct blows and often it is rapid changes in direction of the head that cause the most significant injuries. For example, any boxer will tell you that a punch which causes the head to rapidly rotate is more likely to knock someone unconscious than a straight punch to the head that does not cause the head to move.

The initial injury to the brain caused by a traumatic event, i.e. the bruising, bleeding, and stretching of the brain tissue, is known as the primary injury. Given the almost infinite variation in how the brain can be squashed, stretched, twisted, and distorted during trauma, the extent of these primary injuries is highly variable between individuals. This primary injury is dependent on the exact mechanics of how the traumatic force is applied to the head as well as individual factors such as neck strength, whether the individual is restrained or wearing a helmet and so on. Due to these subtle differences, seemingly similar traumatic forces can produce very different injuries between individuals. We have all heard stories or, perhaps, know someone who has walked away from a highspeed car accident with only cuts and bruises, yet I have also seen individuals with bleeding in the brain caused by a seemingly innocuous blow to the head.

After the initial injury, further damage to the brain tissue can be caused by numerous other processes. These include swelling in the brain, reduced blood flow to areas of the brain not initially injured, disruption to normal brain cell functions and damage from toxic substances released at the time of injury from damaged cells. These processes can all add to the extent of the initial damage and are collectively known as the secondary injury. Much of the early medical treatment is aimed at minimising this secondary injury to prevent any further loss of brain tissue and minimise the overall volume of damaged brain tissue.

In addition to these primary and secondary injury processes, people's body's respond to injury in different ways and it soon becomes apparent that traumatic brain injury is a very broad term. It is not a single, uniform entity; rather it is a highly complex process dependent upon the interaction between the nature and the severity of the injury and the individual who suffers it. No two injuries or resulting problems are the same. This is an important point to understand when recovering from brain trauma because comparisons to other people are often unhelpful.

After a minor head injury, the brain often looks completely normal on a CT scan but that does not mean there have not been changes at a level not visible on the scans. A normal scan does not mean that someone will not nor should not have symptoms; in fact, changes on a scan can bear little relation to the severity of symptoms suffered. This variation makes the assessment of people who have suffered a head injury complex and requires careful evaluation of an individual's problems and needs.

Doctors and patients alike often make the mistake of placing too much emphasis on the imaging of the brain. An early scan is useful to make sure there is no significant bleeding that requires urgent treatment, but too much is often placed on the use of a scan later on to try and explain ongoing symptoms. It feels intuitive that if you have damaged your brain a 'picture' of it (as achieved via a CT or MRI scan) should show you that damage. A normal scan must surely mean there is no significant injury. To some extent this is true, it is always more reassuring to have a normal scan as they are very good at identifying large areas of bruising or bleeding in the brain. However, when the brain is shaken within the skull the brain cells (neurons) can be stretched, pulled and injured. Given the fact these brain cells are tiny (0.004mm to 0.1mm) and a standard MRI scan has a resolution of 1mm^3, these scans clearly cannot 'see' evidence of injury at the level of the neuron. More sophisticated imaging methods can identify evidence of injury at a scale not detected on normal scans and so it is wrong to conclude that a normal brain scan equals no brain injury.

In addition to structural injury to the cells within the brain, other processes occurring after injury can affect how the brain works. To understand this, it can be useful to think about how other areas of the body respond to an injury as this is something we have all experienced and can relate to. If we bang our arm we will initially experience some localised pain. If the bang was hard enough, the area will swell, become hot, tender and a bruise will develop. This process involves the release of substances from damaged cells in the area of injury, but other substances necessary for aiding the healing process are also released into the area of injury. This can also happen in the injured brain. Importantly, the brain requires a very carefully balanced chemical environment to function normally and therefore, even if the brain cells themselves are not damaged, a disruption to their chemical environment can hinder their ability to work normally. To understand this better, let us think about how the brain works and how even basic brain functions might be disrupted if the brain cells are working sub-optimally:

At a simplistic level, the brain works by sending electrical signals along individual brain cells. The brain cells themselves are a bit like telephone cables or electrical wires; they are mostly long and thin and travel between different areas of the brain. The individual cells 'talk' to each other at synapses where chemicals are released between the cells to continue the electrical signals. For the brain to work properly, the signals passing along and between individual cells must be highly co-ordinated. The process of sending electrical signals is dependent on the chemical environment both inside and outside the brain cells and this is carefully regulated by various complex mechanisms present on the brain cells, in the space between them, and in the blood vessels that supply the brain with oxygen and nutrients. Even a minor impact to the brain can lead to a release of substances that may disrupt this carefully balanced environment, thereby hindering normal brain cell function.

To understand how this may cause problems, let us think about the processes required to carry out a simple task like having a conversation. During a conversation, the sounds generated by the other person are transmitted to the brain via our ears. The sounds are turned into electrical signals, these signals are sent to the brain to make sense of the sounds. Once processed, these signals are sent onward to another part of the brain to digest the information received, then sent further to the area responsible for considering a response and then on to the area involved in generating a speech output by triggering the muscles required to create an appropriate speech response. All of this happens in a fraction of a second. Any delay or disruption to this process will upset the careful co-ordination of the brain. Therefore, if the brain is not able to function normally due to a disruption in its environment, processes that we take for granted, like having a conversation, become more effortful. Errors, tiredness and fatigue are common complaints that people experience in this situation due to the brain struggling. In addition, as the brain finds it harder to work, concentration levels drop as the brain tries to "conserve" its energy. This can be perceived as a problem with memory, as people often report forgetting recent conversations or bits of information. Rather than being a memory problem as such, this failure to remember things is because the brain has not been concentrating on those conversations in a bid to preserve energy.

How long does it take to recover from a brain injury?

This is of course a difficult question to answer as it depends on many factors. We will explore the factors that predispose to a prolonged resolution of symptoms in the next section, but it is worth commenting that people's expectations of speed of recovery after a mild head injury are often over-optimistic. This 'over-optimism' is commonly compounded by information provided both by medical professionals and available in books and on the internet. The implication that 'concussion' is a transient short-lived phenomenon commonly results in advice stating all symptoms should resolve within a few days. While this is true for many people and it is certainly important to remain optimistic (assuming you will be left with persistent problems is a sure-fire way of ending up with persistent symptoms!) an unrealistic expectation for recovery can cause problems as well:

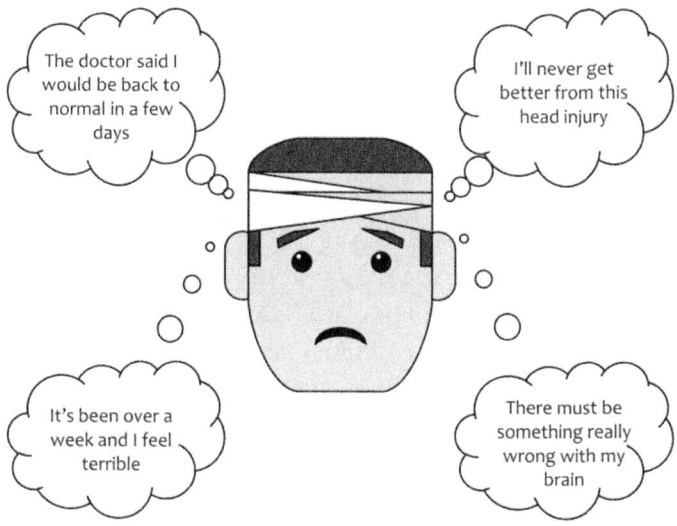

We are all different and, for some of us, symptoms can take many weeks or months to improve. However, if symptoms go on for longer than a couple of weeks it is worth seeking medical help as we know that early intervention can help considerably. As we will go on to discuss in the next section there are many reasons why symptoms can persist. Some have a simple fix given correct and early intervention and, just as importantly, it is very rare for persisting symptoms to be an indicator that the brain cannot eventually get better.

It is also important to make clear the distinction between having persistent symptoms following a minor head injury and the longer-term risks of repeated minor head injuries. There has been a great deal of medical, media and public interest in the risks of developing progressive brain disease (a type of dementia called chronic traumatic encephalopathy or CTE) after repeated minor head injuries and much of this interest has been generated in a sporting context. We shall discuss this further in the section "What are the long-term consequences?" but, in the rare situations when CTE develops, this occurs *many* years after the head injuries themselves and it is important to emphasise that the late development of CTE is very different from and not related to the persistent symptoms that someone can experience after a minor head injury or concussion. These persistent symptoms are not risk factors themselves for the development of CTE.

We shall now look at what factors can lead to persistent symptoms in some people and then discuss what we know (and do not know) about chronic traumatic encephalopathy.

Why do some people have persistent symptoms?

This is a complex question and, unsurprisingly, there is no single, simple answer to it. Many factors interplay and potentially contribute to a prolongation of symptoms, making it important to identify the cause – or combination of causes – in any one individual with persistent symptoms.

Historically, persistent symptoms after a minor head injury were viewed as a purely 'psychological' phenomenon. However, we now know that there are many biological causes (e.g. precipitation or exacerbation of migraine, damage to the balance apparatus in the inner ear) that can contribute to prolonging symptoms in an individual. These 'biological' factors will often interact with 'psychological' factors and one frequently exacerbates the other. For example, damage to the balance apparatus in the inner ear will cause exceptionally unpleasant feelings of vertigo and imbalance. This commonly triggers anxiety and understandable distress that these highly disabling symptoms will last for ever and that they are signs of significant damage to the brain. Therefore, given the array of potential causes for persistent symptoms and their very different treatment options, a clear assessment of the reasons why an individual is suffering prolonged symptoms is vital to directing appropriate treatment for that individual.

It can be useful to separate the causes for the development of persistent symptoms into pre-injury, injury and post-injury factors. Recognition of these issues helps patients and doctors to understand why symptoms may not have improved and, although it may not always be possible to change all contributing factors – personality type is an example – it is nevertheless surprisingly beneficial for someone to realise that over-anxiety or some other personality influence is playing a part in prolonging their head injury symptoms.

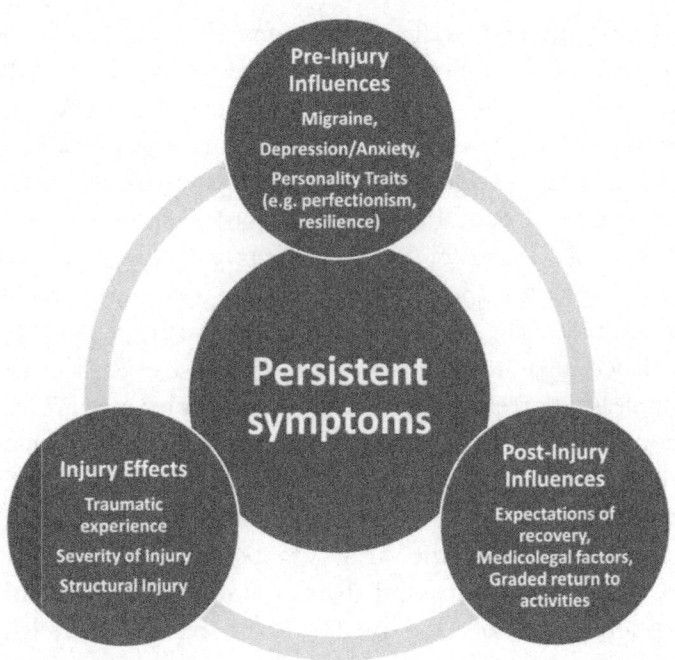

Injury factors:

In terms of the injury factors, the severity of the injury itself and the degree of injury to brain structures is important. For example, if you damage the balance apparatus in your inner ear, you may develop prolonged feelings of dizziness and vertigo. Equally the psychological trauma of the event that caused the head injury will influence the risk of developing psychological and psychiatric symptoms including anxiety and post-traumatic stress disorder. People often underestimate the trauma of an event and downplay the effect that it has had on them psychologically, but it is important to recognise this and to seek professional help if you feel that psychological issues like anxiety or depression are affecting you.

Pre-injury factors:

A great deal of research has focused on pre-injury risk factors that increase the likelihood of the development of persistent symptoms after a mild head injury.

Certain personality traits predispose individuals to an increased risk of developing persistent symptoms. We all have unique personality traits and behaviours, some of us are more optimistic, others pessimistic, some are naturally anxious whilst others are carefree. Recognising what kind of person we are is important in all aspects of life and will also play into the risks of developing persistent symptoms after a head injury. People more prone to anxiety, pessimism and those with perfectionist traits appear to be more at risk of developing persistent symptoms. In addition to our personality type, individuals with prior mental health problems, previous brain injuries or neurological problems are also at greater risk. Migraine is a particularly important case. Migraine is surprisingly common – around 1 in 7 people suffer migraines – and for those with a prior history of migraine, the risk of developing a worse headache after even a mild head injury is incredibly high, with up to 50% reporting a worse headache even a year after the injury. For these people, prompt treatment is important as the likelihood of symptoms' resolving on their own is unlikely. It is important to be clear, however, that these factors do not mean you *will* have prolonged symptoms, they are just factors that make prolonged symptoms *more* likely.

Post-injury factors:

Finally, there are certain post-injury factors that can perpetuate post-head injury symptoms. Over optimistic expectations for recovery can sometimes lead to a perpetuation of symptoms. If someone feels that they should be better within a few days (they may even have been told this by a health professional) but is still experiencing symptoms beyond this time, the mismatch between *actual* recovery and *expected* recovery is very good at causing psychological distress that itself prolongs the symptoms even more – in fact, possibly even after the brain has recovered fully.

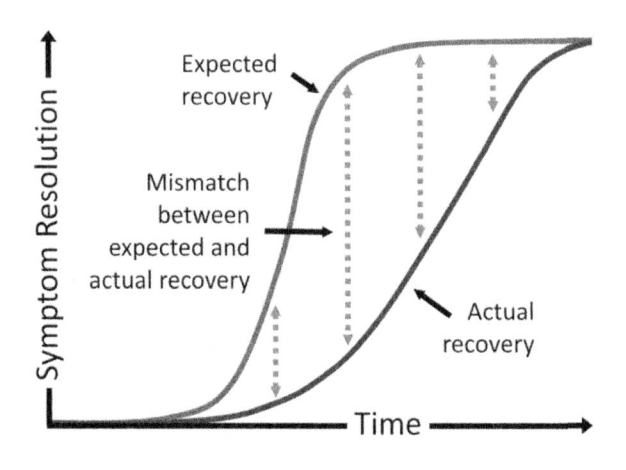

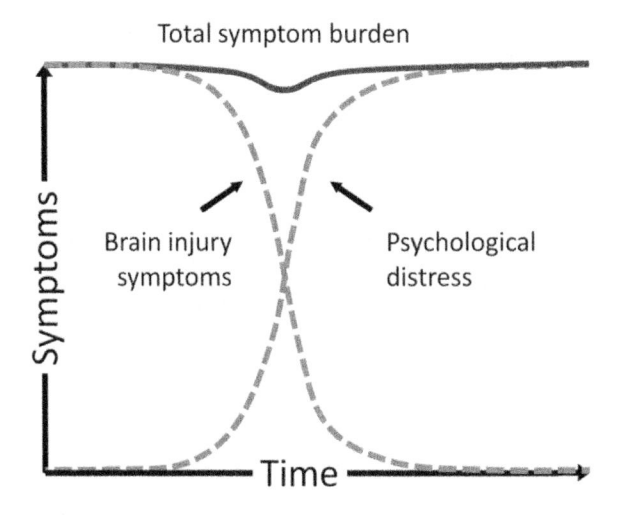

This has been proposed as one of the main causes of prolongation of symptoms after a minor head injury. Initially, biological factors are the main cause of symptoms (i.e. brain swelling and chemical disruption causing headache and associated symptoms) but, as these resolve, psychological factors predominate and lead to a persistence of symptoms. This is probably true to an extent in many patients and maybe the sole reason for persistence in some. However, quite commonly there is also an underlying biological factor (e.g. migraine) in this complex mix, whose biological effects succeed in exacerbating the psychological distress experienced by someone who feels they should be getting better and is not.

These examples illustrate just how complex and interactive many factors – both biological and psychological – are in enabling the persistence of debilitating symptoms after head injury. Because of these complexities, and because everyone is different, it follows that individual assessment is vital in these cases and included in this approach is the central need for exploration and treatment of underlying biological factors. These are not only important contributors to symptomatology themselves but are also powerful compounders of any psychological factors that may co-exist. This melting-pot has even more potential for complication as psychological disturbance may mask any biological contribution, preventing their recognition and hence treatment. Under these circumstances, psychological treatments alone are highly unlikely to be successful unless co-existing biological factors are also addressed.

Another factor to consider is the psychological impact of the cause of the injury. Head injuries frequently occur in the context of accidents or sometimes from purposeful attacks where another person is to blame. The ensuing anger and bitterness, or perceived injustice is another common cause of psychological distress and prolongation of symptoms.

Additionally, legal processes are recognised to perpetuate symptoms. Rather than this being an active decision to exaggerate or 'make-up' symptoms by the injured party for financial gain, it is most commonly caused by the protracted way legal processes tend to proceed with the resulting stress and the continued reminder of the incident for the injured party. This is not a recommendation to not pursue a legal case, but it is important to highlight the potential impact it can have and to recognise this in the context of prolonged symptoms.

Medications can also sometimes have a negative impact. It is not uncommon to be prescribed a variety of pain relief medications after an injury, particularly if there are also injuries to other parts of the body. These medications are important in the first few weeks after trauma and are unlikely to cause a problem at this stage. However, it is not uncommon to find people on strong pain medications months after the injury. Most of these medications have potent effects on the brain; they can affect our thinking, make us feel dizzy, disrupt sleep, and can even lead to persistent 'medication overuse' headache (see Headache section). Re-assessing the need for pain medication is therefore important at all stages and unnecessary medications should be weaned off and stopped.

Finally, the way we approach the recovery period can affect our risk of perpetuating symptoms. Sometimes I see people who suffer a head injury on a Sunday and by the Monday they are back at work at 7am, working 12-hour days and exercising and socialising throughout the weekend. Invariably, these people collapse in a heap after a few weeks with a plethora of symptoms as the brain has been unable to recover. Equally, I see people who become so concerned by their injury and the risk of exacerbating it that they stay in bed or on the sofa, resting for weeks on end. This leads to deconditioning and they struggle to get back to their previous life as everything seems exhausting. This can perpetuate the idea that the brain has not fully recovered and that more rest is required when the opposite is true. Therefore, during the recovery period it is important to walk a fine line, being careful not to overdo things whilst also making sure you are not doing too little so that you decondition. It is a little bit like exercise; if you go to the gym and do not get out of breath you will not improve your fitness levels, equally if you have never run further than a few hundred metres, embarking on a marathon without proper training is likely to end in your collapsing in a heap.

What are the long-term consequences?

Overall, the long-term prognosis after a single minor head injury is extremely good with most people making a full recovery. Nearly half of us will suffer some form of head injury in our lives and clearly most of us do not suffer persistent problems nor do we develop future neurological complications.

At this stage, it is important to be clear about the distinction between:

- Persistent problems that develop at the time of the head injury, or soon after, and do not improve.

and

- Complications such as epilepsy or dementia that may develop many years *after* the injury.

We have discussed the factors associated with the risk of developing persistent symptoms above; here we shall discuss the risk of future complications including second-impact syndrome, epilepsy, dementia and whether a head injury will shorten our lifespan. Before we embark on these issues, I want to emphasise very strongly that, after a single mild head injury, the risk of developing future problems is **very** low.

Second-impact syndrome:

First, I want to discuss the so-called "second-impact syndrome". This syndrome was first recognised in the 1970s, with rare cases of people dying from catastrophic brain swelling after a relatively minor head injury. In these cases, it was noted that the individuals had suffered a preceding minor head injury prior to receiving a second injury that led to severe brain swelling and death. Second-impact syndrome is a slightly controversial topic, as the evidence for a preceding head injury is often limited. The catastrophic swelling may instead be a very rare complication of an isolated injury and the presence of a previous injury may not be of relevance. The most important thing to stress about second-impact syndrome is that it is *incredibly* rare (may be one or two cases a year). Assuming the initial injury is an important event and can predispose to a second catastrophic event, it adds support to the sensible view that full recovery from a head injury is important before considering return to an activity that risks exposure to a further head injury such as a contact sport (see 'Return to contact sports' section for how to manage this).

Epilepsy:

A single mild head injury does seem to slightly increase our risk of developing epilepsy. This increased risk is actually very small (about 0.1% absolute risk over the first year, or 1 extra person in 1000 developing epilepsy) and returns to the normal background risk of developing epilepsy (about 0.05% risk per year, or 5 people in every 10,000) within a few years. Developing post-traumatic epilepsy depends on many factors, not least the severity of the head injury itself. To put this in context, the description of a "mild head injury" has a broad compass, ranging from a minor bang on the head without loss of consciousness to being knocked out for a few minutes and confused for several hours afterwards. Additional factors such as our genetics and lifestyle also influence the risk of developing epilepsy and for some people a truly minor injury may be enough to precipitate epilepsy if they already had an increased risk through these other factors. For most people, however, a minor head injury is unlikely to have a significant impact on our risk of developing epilepsy.

Dementia:

The risk of developing dementia after minor head injuries has gained a great deal of public, media and scientific interest recently. This is obviously a major concern given the prevalence of minor head injuries, with half of us suffering some form of head injury during our lives. In addition, it raises important questions about the potential danger posed by sports, jobs or pastimes that confer a greater risk of suffering a head injury. However, there has been a great deal of confusion around this subject. It is important to clarify what we mean by the term dementia in this context, what we know (and do not know) so far and to be mindful of the potential dangers created by focussing on this particular aspect, especially if other treatable issues are missed.

For most people, the term dementia implies a progressive loss of brain function that occurs in older people and ultimately results in a loss of independence and ability to care for oneself. Most people relate dementia to impairments in memory, i.e. not being able to remember recent events or recognise people, principally because this is the commonest presenting feature in the most common form of dementia, namely Alzheimer's disease.

Although this perception of dementia is correct to a degree, it is more accurately defined as a syndrome in which there is a disturbance of higher brain functions that impacts on someone's ability to carry out their normal activities of daily living. It is more common in older people but it can happen at any age. Higher brain functions include processes such as memory, learning, language, decision-making, concentrating, recognising emotions in others and judgement. Although most causes of dementia lead to a progressive decline in these abilities, 'fixed' or 'static' impairments are also considered under the dementia label if they are long-standing. This latter point is most relevant in the context of a traumatic brain injury, especially a severe brain injury that has caused permanent brain damage. This may result in a long-lasting impairment of one or more of the above brain functions. However, unlike other forms of dementia such as Alzheimer's disease, this impairment may not necessarily worsen over time but can still be considered a type of dementia using the above definition.

Although severe traumatic brain injuries can lead to permanent impairments in brain function that fulfil the definition for "dementia", the risk of an isolated mild head injury causing a permanent impairment in brain function that affects daily living, and hence would be classified as a dementia, is very low. It is important to reiterate, that in this context we are referring to an impairment in brain function caused by damage to the brain at *the time of* the injury and persisting for a long time afterwards. It is also important to highlight that there are many other reasons for an impairment, or perceived impairment, in brain functioning after a head injury that are **not** caused by a dementia. Anxiety, low mood and pain will all disrupt our brain's ability to function normally as it is overwhelmed by these other factors. In addition, a mild head injury is a common trigger for so-called functional cognitive symptoms (see Chapter 4 "Difficulties with memory, concentration and speed of thinking" for further details). Functional cognitive symptoms are common but under-recognised, most people have heard of dementia but surprisingly few have heard of functional cognitive symptoms despite it being common. Functional cognitive symptoms are defined as a problem with memory or concentration due to the brain not working or functioning as we expect it to, they are **not** caused by disease or damage to the brain – i.e. they are not due to dementia. I will discuss how functional cognitive symptoms can easily develop following a mild head injury and treatment options further in Chapter 4.

Separate to this 'fixed' impairment of brain function that develops at the time of the brain injury and persists, brain injuries can increase the risk of developing a progressive form of dementia that develops years after the injury. It is this aspect that has gained much of the recent media attention as it has been shown to occur in individuals who have suffered repeated minor head injuries. This has been most closely examined in the context of contact sports such as American football, boxing and soccer, but any cause of repeated minor head injuries has been implicated. Despite this recent media attention, we have known for nearly a hundred years that repeated minor head injuries increases the risk of developing dementia. Boxers were recognised to suffer progressive impairments of brain function even after stopping boxing. This was termed "punch-drunk syndrome" and later "dementia pugilistica". Since the turn of this century, there has been increasing recognition that any cause of repeated minor head injury can predispose to this risk of developing a progressive form of dementia that is distinct from other forms of dementia when the brain in these individuals is examined under a microscope. This type of dementia has been termed "chronic traumatic encephalopathy" ('chronic' means lasting for a long time or constantly recurring and 'encephalopathy' means a disease affecting the functioning of the brain). It has become particularly noted in American football players and other contact sports and it is increasingly clear that repeated head injuries increase the risk of developing a progressive form of dementia in the future.

However, we do not know how common CTE is, we do not know how many or how severe the head injuries must be and, importantly, this is a condition that, at the current time, can only be diagnosed *after* death at post-mortem when the brain tissue is examined under a microscope. The risk of developing CTE seems to be associated with the number of head injuries suffered and, as in many other diseases, there is also likely to be a genetic component that means some people are at greater risk than others of developing this condition. There have been attempts to characterise the symptoms of CTE in life, but these overlap with many other conditions (including depression). Neither are there any clever tests at the moment that are specific for CTE and so it is not possible to accurately determine the presence of this condition in a living person.

A single severe brain injury also appears to increase the risk of developing a future progressive dementia years after the injury. However, an isolated mild head injury does not appear to increase the risk of developing a progressive dementia later in life.

In summary, there is clearly a link between repeated minor head injuries and the risk of developing a dementia. However, it is important to keep this in context and to recognise that there is much we do not know. Playing sport is incredibly beneficial at many levels and a recent study showed that ex-soccer players had a lower mortality rate in general (from heart disease etc) but also an increased risk of developing dementia, highlighting the potential pros and cons of playing sports. It is important that we make sports (and other aspects of life) safer and limit head injuries, whilst recognising that a healthy lifestyle is also important.

Life expectancy:

There are conflicting studies showing a potential association between mild head injury and long-term mortality. One study showed elevated long-term death rates in individuals who had been admitted to hospital with a mild traumatic brain injury. Other large studies have not found this association. Overall, it is unlikely that a single minor head injury will lead to reduced lifespan.

Finally, it is important to recognise that there is no clear cut-off between minor and more severe head injuries. Instead, there is a continuum, and the risk of future problems is related to the severity of the injury. In addition to the severity of the injury itself there are other factors that increase the risk of long-term problems. Of these, genetics and pre-existing health conditions are the biggest contributors we know about. For example, someone with a predisposition to epilepsy may need only a relatively minor head injury to trigger epilepsy, whereas someone with a severe head injury may never suffer seizures if their other genetic and lifestyle factors are protective against seizures.

How can I get better?

We will discuss specific symptoms later but there are a few general strategies that can help to accelerate recovery and prevent continuation or worsening of symptoms.

The first point to make is that it is *extremely* rare to develop new, serious complications more than a day after a minor head injury. It is not uncommon for symptoms to change or worsen over the first few days, but this is normally in the context of a trigger (e.g. performing a task requiring concentration or physical activity) and is usually short-lived. However, if you are concerned that your symptoms are worsening, and certainly if you develop any of the following, you should return to an emergency department immediately for assessment:

- Any loss of consciousness or collapse
- Unable to wake or severe drowsiness
- Balance problems or difficulty walking
- Vision, speaking or hearing problems
- Clear fluid coming from mouth or ears
- Weakness in arms or legs
- Severe headache not relieved by painkillers
- Vomiting

Rest and graded return:

There is some debate regarding how long we should rest after a head injury. There is good evidence in most medical situations from broken legs to severe brain injuries that early rehabilitation is beneficial. It is surprising how quickly the body deconditions if not being used and this applies equally to the brain. Early rehabilitation is vital in getting both body and brain back to normal as quickly as possible. It is reasonable to rest for 24-48 hours after a minor head injury if needed. It is then important to start doing things, even if this is just gentle exercise such as walking. Doing nothing will certainly delay recovery.

Avoiding excess sensory stimuli can be helpful early on. Bright lights and loud noises can produce sensory overload and the brain may struggle to process these external inputs. Avoiding computer screens is often recommended to avoid sensory overload on the brain and remember that bright electronic screens can also disrupt our normal body clock, especially if viewed at night-time. The brain is particularly sensitive to disruptions during this period and even if you found it easy to use your computer late at night and then fall straight to sleep before the injury, you are likely to find this much harder afterwards.

After a brief period of rest, all aspects of brain functioning then need to be gradually increased, including physical exercise, tasks requiring concentration and exposure to sensory inputs. Only you can judge the speed at which this can be done, but as a rule of thumb, if life is not getting back on track within two weeks it is worth seeking medical help as early intervention will reduce the risk of developing persistent problems. To be clear, symptoms can (and often do) last longer than a couple of weeks after a minor head injury. If they have not fully resolved by 2 weeks it does **not** mean you have permanently damaged your brain, rather seeking help sooner rather than later can help if there are other factors that can be treated (e.g. migraine or BPPV – see Headache and Dizziness sections).

Do not panic!

Let us consider a sprained ankle as an analogy. If we rested a sprained ankle for 24-48 hours and then decided to run 5km a day for a week we would not be too surprised if we came hobbling in at the end of each run (even assuming we could finish the whole 5km anyway!). If at the end of that week our ankle had swollen and it was more painful to walk, we would probably think we had over-done it, we would rest it, ice it and decide we had been a bit stupid. We would then (hopefully!) decide to build up our exercise gradually over the next few weeks, stretch our ankle and look after it. We probably would not think we had a major ankle injury that would never get better, buy a pair of crutches and not use our ankle properly for several weeks leading to the ankle's stiffening up and delaying recovery.

This may seem obvious, but this is exactly what tends to happen after a head injury, but why? People often rest for a day and then launch straight back into normal life after a minor head injury. This can lead to a major worsening of symptoms and is sometimes referred to as a 'boom and bust' phenomenon. It seems obvious that running and walking will inflame an injured ankle but most of us do not consider how much work our brain does on a daily basis, even for seemingly simple processes. The brain uses 20% of the body's energy yet makes up just 2% of the body's weight; it is therefore easy to overload an injured brain that has not had the time to heal properly.

The brain controls and determines how we walk, talk, feel, think, and process information; therefore, if it is not working at full capacity, we can feel like our world is turned upside down. It is therefore not hard to see how we can catastrophize in this situation as there is no obvious swollen ankle to attribute to our difficulties and it is easy to believe there may be a significant underlying brain injury to explain why we are unable to function normally. Just as with a sprained ankle, the worst thing to do is to then do nothing and decondition the brain – instead, we should concentrate on looking after our brain (optimise sleep, eat healthily and gentle exercise) and adopt a more gradual graded return to mental activities.

Pacing strategies

To help with this, it can be useful to consider certain pacing strategies early on while your brain is recovering and is not as productive as normal. Try to plan your day into manageable chunks and arrange breaks when you can let your brain rest and do not spend this time in front of a computer or TV screen! During these breaks try using meditation or mindfulness techniques. There are plenty of apps and online resources that can help you with this.

For most people, this period of pacing will be relatively short-lived. After a few days to a week, you should find that you are almost back to normal. If it is lasting longer than a couple of weeks, then again it is worth seeking help to rule out other causes for the ongoing fatigue such as mood problems.

Tell people around you

The increased media attention regarding head injuries has improved most people's understanding that its effects can be significant and not always visible. There is no obligation to tell your work or those around you, but in nearly all cases sharing your problem does prove to be helpful. Rarely do I encounter people who have had difficulty with their work colleagues or employers after they have informed them of their head injury. Not telling your work and subsequently having to take time off or making errors if you are struggling to concentrate are far greater risks. In most situations it is helpful to let your work know, agree a graded return plan and even supervision initially if errors in your work have the potential for serious consequences.

People around you should also know. Irritability is one of the most common symptoms following head injury and is often a result of fatigue. If those around you are aware, they will be more understanding and can help with tasks to allow you to recover.

Treat the treatables

The general mantra concerning recovery from a minor head injury is "things will improve with time". This is commonly the case, but as we will discover below, many symptoms can have particular causes that need specific treatments and time does not necessarily treat them. We will go into more detail in the relevant sections but, for example, people who suffer migraines prior to the head injury are at high risk of developing worse or persistent headaches after a minor head injury and therefore warrant prompt treatment. Damage to the balance apparatus in the inner ear is also common and there are specific treatments and manoeuvres that can correct this immediately in certain cases thereby avoiding prolonged, unpleasant symptoms of unsteadiness and vertigo. These issues are examples of why seeking help from your doctor after two weeks if you are not better is advised.

Be aware of the effect of medications

Certain medications are needed after an injury. If you also suffered injuries to other parts of your body, you may well need painkillers. In the short term these can be important to alleviate pain and to aid rest and sleep. However, it is important to remember that they often have other effects including impairing our thinking, disrupting our sleep, and making us feel sick. Many of these symptoms are similar to those attributed to "post-concussion syndrome" and weaning off unnecessary medications is an important process before ascribing symptoms to the brain injury itself.

Prolonged use of painkillers can also lead to a 'medication-overuse headache'. A medication-overuse headache is a dull, constant headache that is present most days or part of every day. Only people prone to headaches tend to develop this problem, generally speaking those with a previous history of migraines or a family history of migraines. They can develop if a susceptible individual takes a painkiller (such as paracetamol, ibuprofen or codeine) more than 2 to 3 times a week for several weeks. It is easy to see how these may develop after a head injury; head injuries typically precipitate or exacerbate headaches, especially in those prone to headaches, leading to an increased use of painkillers, and ultimately the generation of a medication-overuse headache. This can result in a vicious cycle, as withdrawing the medication can worsen the headache in the short-term, making it very difficult to refrain from taking further painkillers. The only way to treat this type of headache is to withdraw the medication and it may need help from your doctor if you are struggling to do so on your own.

Doctors like to prescribe medications, often these are helpful and can alleviate troublesome symptoms, but they can also have unintended consequences. For example, it is not uncommon to be prescribed an anti-sickness tablet for prolonged symptoms of dizziness or vertigo. We will discuss this further in the dedicated section on dizziness, but if the vertigo is due to injury to the balance apparatus in the inner ear, taking these medications for more than a few days can hinder rehabilitation of this system and lead to persistent feelings of dizziness. There are also potential problems with sleeping tablets; these can help for a few days, but prolonged use can disrupt our natural sleep pattern, impair our quality of sleep and worsen sleep in the longer term.

Finally, many people enjoy an alcoholic drink every now and then. It is important to recognise that alcohol is a brain toxin and affects brain function, something that all of us are aware of when we see people slurring and stumbling if they have drunk too much. With a recovering brain, you will find that much less alcohol is needed to affect your brain function. It is therefore wise to avoid alcohol until symptoms resolve and to recognise that even after symptoms are better, you may find alcohol affects you more than previously for some time after a head injury.

PART 2:
Symptoms after a concussion

1. Headache

Headaches are the most common and often the most problematic symptom experienced after a head injury. If we banged our arm or leg, we would not be surprised if it hurt afterwards and therefore it makes sense that headaches are common after a head injury. However, there can be different causes for a headache following a head injury that need to be considered as treatments can vary.

Understandably, people are often concerned that a headache is the sign of a serious problem in the brain, such as bleeding or permanent brain injury. This is *very* rarely the case after a minor head injury and development of a migraine-like headache is by far the most common cause of a post-traumatic headache. However, awareness of symptoms and signs of a potentially serious cause for the headache is important. The presence of any of the symptoms in the box below warrants an assessment by a healthcare professional:

> **Headache symptoms after a mild head injury that warrant a review by a healthcare professional**
>
> - Worsening/severe headache not responding to painkillers
> - Clear fluid coming from nose or ears (potential for fluid leaking from around the brain or spine)
> - Headache worse on lying and resolved on standing or worse in the morning (possibility of raised pressure in and around the brain)
> - Headache worse on standing and resolved on lying (possibility of reduced pressure in and around the brain)
> - Any weakness or numbness of the limbs

As many as 9 out of 10 people will experience a headache after a mild head injury but, perhaps surprisingly, between 3 and 5 out of 10 people report a new or worse headache even 1 year after an injury. People with a prior history of migraines (or a family history of migraines) are especially at risk of developing a new or worse headache. Presumably, this is because their genetic makeup makes them more susceptible to suffering headaches and are therefore more at risk of worsening headaches after a traumatic brain injury.

Post-traumatic headaches are not a trivial issue and can cause significant disability. About a third of people suffering a post-traumatic headache are unable to return to their previous level of work 3 months after the injury. Therefore, rather than considering a post-traumatic headache to be just one of the many symptoms of a 'post-concussion syndrome' that should 'just get better', it is important to assess the cause of the headache and treat appropriately to prevent the risk of persistent symptoms and their impact on daily life.

Post-traumatic headache is defined as a new headache (or worse headache if headaches were a pre-existing condition) that develops within 7 days of a head injury. This is not a particularly helpful definition as it does not help to guide treatment, does not recognise the different types of post-traumatic headache and does not acknowledge that it is not uncommon to develop headaches even a few months after a head injury.

Therefore, when treating a post-traumatic headache, we first aim to exclude a serious cause and then try to determine the type of headache suffered to help guide which treatment may work. As mentioned previously, there are no proven treatments for post-traumatic headache per se, rather a selection of treatments known to work for other headache disorders that we presume may also work for post-traumatic headache.

Causes of post-traumatic headache:

The cause of post-traumatic headache is not fully understood, and several theories of causation have been proposed. As the brain is responsible for creating our perception of pain, disruption to this "pain generating" system because of trauma is one proposed mechanism. Release of toxic substances and ongoing inflammation in the brain is another suggested idea. Currently, there are trials looking at whether specific treatments targeting these mechanisms may be of benefit in treating post-traumatic headache. As there are no specific, proven treatments for post-traumatic headache we tend to characterise the 'type' of headache and treat in a way similar to that we would use to treat that type of headache if it were not due to trauma. Using this approach, migraine-like headache is the most common type of post-traumatic headache, followed by tension-type headache, neck injury related headaches and then various rarer types.

Migraine:

Most post-traumatic headaches have similar features to migraine headaches. Migraine-type headaches last several hours (up to a few days), can be on one side of the head or both, are often throbbing or pulsating in nature, are exacerbated by routine activities like walking, are associated with nausea and/or vomiting and are aggravated by bright lights and loud noises.

For those suffering migraine-like post-traumatic headaches it is important to be aware that migraine is not *just* a headache but is instead a brain disorder. Migraines have many other associated symptoms including nausea, vomiting, dizziness, light sensitivity, noise sensitivity, irritability and 'brain fog'. You can see from this list that migraine causes similar symptoms to those classed as post-concussion related symptoms. For people who have suffered migraines prior to their injury, these associated symptoms are not a surprise but for people without experience of migraine headaches this multitude of associated symptoms can cause significant anxiety and concern that there is a worrying underlying cause pointing to a serious problem with their brain. Therefore, recognition of a post-traumatic migraine-like headache and treatment can help many post-head injury symptoms. In fact, in some cases, migraine may be the only cause of ongoing symptoms.

Tension-type headache:

The second most common type of post-traumatic headache is a tension-type headache. Tension-type headaches are very common outside of the context of a head injury. They are typically on both sides of the head and feel like a squeezing or pressing type pain. There can be tenderness around the scalp but there should not be any of the migrainous qualities detailed above such as nausea, vomiting or excessive pain. They are commonly not as severe as a migraine-type headache and usual resolve with simple painkillers. Massage and acupuncture may also help, but if the headaches are persistent further treatments from your doctor may be required.

Headache related to neck injury:

Injury to the neck can cause headache. Commonly these headaches radiate from the neck up the back of the head and are triggered or exacerbated by neck movements. The neck is commonly stiff with restricted movements and there is often tenderness of the neck muscles. These headaches can be limited to one side of the head and do not necessarily need to spread up from the neck. Interestingly, these headaches can be associated with other features such as nausea and dislike of bright lights and loud noises. Massage, acupuncture and physiotherapy for the neck issues can be successful at treating this type of headache.

Other headache types:

There are various other rarer headache types that can develop. Occasionally, pain from the nerves around the head and neck can be triggered following a traumatic injury. These are brief, intense, electric-shock type pains that can spread over the head.

For all headache types, the general treatments below still apply but if ineffective, assessment by a suitable healthcare professional is recommended.

Headache treatments:

Detailed assessment by a healthcare professional may be needed but there are a few simple steps that anyone can take to help treat their headaches.

First, make sure you are not taking too many painkillers. This may seem odd, but regular use of painkillers can *cause* a persistent headache, a so-called medication overuse headache. This type of headache typically occurs if you take regular painkillers for more than 15 days a month for at least 3 months. The headache itself is often quite featureless, never really goes away with painkillers and is of a moderate intensity. In this situation it is important to **stop** the pain medications. This may lead to a worsening of headaches for a couple of weeks, but they will then improve. If you find it too difficult to stop the medications due to worsening pain or the need for painkillers for another reason, then you will need to seek medical help to assist you in this process.

There are some general measures anyone can do to help improve headaches, these mainly relate to migraine-type headaches, but as mentioned this is the most common type of post-traumatic headache and, unless there is a clear alternative cause, these simple measures are worth a try.

1. Ensure regularity of your daily routine. This is particularly important with regards to sleep as sleep deprivation is a key cause of migraine exacerbation.

61

Other aspects of the daily routine, including meals, should also be kept to a regular schedule.

2. Maintaining a healthy lifestyle with exercise and diet. This may sound obvious, but it is surprisingly effective. Regular headaches can make exercise difficult (especially soon after a head injury) and vigorous exercise may not be possible and may even exacerbate the headache, but even getting out for a walk in the sunshine is a helpful step.

3. Certain foods and environments can worsen migrainous headaches. Common examples are alcohol, chocolate, caffeine, bright lights, loud noises, and places with lots of sensory stimuli (e.g. train stations or supermarkets). It is therefore best to avoid these early on if possible.

4. Acupuncture or massage therapy may help some people, particularly if there is associated neck muscle pain and both are safe.

5. Certain supplements including magnesium, riboflavin (Vitamin B2) and co-enzyme Q10 have some evidence for efficacy in migraine. They are all safe if taken as directed although there is no evidence for use after a head injury. These can be bought from a health food store.

In addition to these non-medication measures, simple over-the-counter painkillers can be helpful. The ones with best efficacy are aspirin and ibuprofen. However, there are a couple of rules to follow to prevent harm. First, be aware of the risk of medication overuse headaches as detailed above. A short course of regular painkillers will not cause a medication overuse headache but regular anti-inflammatory drugs such as these can cause stomach irritation and other side effects. Secondly, ibuprofen and aspirin to treat a headache should be taken at a high dose (e.g. 600mg ibuprofen or 600mg dispersible aspirin), at the onset of the headache and no more regularly than 3 times a week. Commonly, people try to avoid taking painkillers and will therefore often wait to see whether the headache will go by itself. Once it becomes apparent that the headache is not improving, it has become established and these medications become much less effective. I therefore recommend that people take these medications as soon as the headache starts with the aim of aborting it rather than 'waiting and seeing' and running the risk of missing the effective treatment window.

If, despite these simple measures, headaches continue it is recommended to see an appropriate healthcare professional as there are many other potential treatment options available on prescription. The risk of persistent post-traumatic headaches is high and therefore warrants prompt treatment.

Case study:

Jon banged his head whilst making a tackle during a game of rugby. He wasn't knocked out but felt dazed for several minutes afterwards.

He developed a headache that evening that was continuous for 3 weeks. He felt sick, a bit dizzy, was unable to concentrate and disliked bright lights and loud noises.

He tried to return to playing rugby but even running exacerbated his headache and symptoms.

> He was seen in the head injury clinic. His headache and symptoms were consistent with a migraine-like post-traumatic headache. He had never had headaches before but his father and elder sister had migraines.
>
> He was reassured that there was no significant brain injury causing his symptoms and that he probably had a predisposition to migraines. He was given lifestyle advice and recommended to take Riboflavin and Magnesium supplements for several weeks. His symptoms settled and he was able to return to rugby with no problems after a few weeks following a graded return programme.

This case highlights how post-traumatic headaches can cause a multitude of symptoms. It is easy to become despondent that the injury has caused a serious head injury if the symptoms persist.

However, a proper understanding of the cause of the symptoms and following good basic lifestyle advice is often enough to resolve the persistent problems. If not, then there are many medications that can benefit this situation and prompt treatment is recommended. People with a pre-existing history of headaches are particularly at risk but so are those who have family members that suffer with headaches. This is because migraine has a genetic component. Migraine-type headaches are typically worsened by exercise, as highlighted in this case. Therefore, it is possible to get a worsening of symptoms when following a graded return to play. This should not cause undue concern as it is normal, and your doctor can give advice on how best to manage the headache.

2. Anxiety and low mood/depression

Disturbance of mood is very common after a head injury and this is particularly true of anxiety. It is important to remember that the brain is responsible for how we feel; it therefore makes sense that, if the brain has been injured, we are quite likely to experience a disruption in our mood as recovery takes place.

In addition, the event itself may well have been traumatising (for example if due to a car accident or an assault). Furthermore, the subsequent impact on someone's life, for example pain in various sites, disrupted sleep and inability to take part in previous leisure activities, is likely to affect a person's mood. This is often referred to as a 'reactive' mood disorder – i.e. it is a 'reaction' to a life event/situation.

Individuals with a pre-existing history of anxiety or low mood are at increased risk of exacerbating these symptoms after a head injury. If you have suffered with either in the past it is important to monitor your mood and seek treatment promptly if you feel that symptoms are returning.

It can often be hard to recognise the development of anxiety or depressive symptoms; they can develop insidiously and be easily dismissed. It can be helpful to check with friends or family who know you well to see if they have noticed a change in your mood. There are also some physical features that may be apparent such as sleeping more or less, early morning waking, reduced appetite and difficulty concentrating, although as you will notice, these are similar to post-head injury symptoms and therefore difficult to disentangle.

Early recognition and treatment are important to avoid mood problems' becoming a longer-term issue. Having an understanding that these are **normal** reactions after a traumatic event is important. They are not a sign of weakness and not something that can be 'snapped out of'. However, they are treatable if the correct treatment options are utilised.

Simple measures that everyone should take include:

- Regular outdoor exercise. It can often help to set it as a daily task – e.g. 30 minutes fast walk around the park.

- Eating healthily and ensuring sleep is optimised will also improve your mood.

- Other ongoing symptoms, for example persistent headache, need to be addressed, as continuous pain or dizziness are potent instigators of a mood disorder.

- Avoid drugs and medications that will worsen mood. Alcohol in particular is a well-recognised depressant, and the brain is more susceptible to its effects after a head injury.

- Relaxation techniques and 'mindfulness' can be very helpful for anxiety symptoms and there are many Apps and websites that can help guide these treatments.

If, despite these simple measures, symptoms persist you should see your doctor to discuss other treatment possibilities. These include talking therapies such as cognitive behavioural therapy (CBT). In addition, there are many different medications that can help. People are often reluctant to take medications; fear of addiction or requiring lifelong treatment are often cited as reasons. As with any medication, if they can be avoided then they should but if symptoms are causing a problem then medications can be very helpful. They can help to boost the chemicals in the brain that are often disrupted after a head injury and are responsible for controlling our mood. Having this lift in mood can be helpful to engage with talking therapies and addiction and dependence are not a problem if taken correctly under the guidance of your doctor.

Case study:

Mary tripped at work and banged her head on the edge of a step. She was briefly knocked out but rapidly came round. She was assessed in the Emergency Department, had a normal scan of her head and was sent home that day with advice.

For the first week she suffered typical post-traumatic symptoms including headache, dizziness, nausea, fatigue and difficulty concentrating. She went back to work after 10 days but developed a worsening of symptoms with a headache, anxiety, feelings of low mood, difficulty thinking, disrupted sleep and apathy.

> She was seen in the head injury clinic having been signed off work for 3 months due to persistent symptoms. On assessment, she was noted to be very low in mood. She reported suffering anxiety and depression prior to the injury and it was clear that the injury, resultant symptoms and time off work had exacerbated these conditions.
> We discussed the cause of her symptoms, she was referred for psychological therapy and started on an anti-depressant. After 3 months of treatment she began a graded return to work and by 6 months her symptoms had improved and she was working full-time.

Mental health conditions including anxiety and depression are incredibly common. Approximately 1 in 4 people will experience mental health problem each year and many do not seek help or treatment.

A head injury will frequently exacerbate mental health conditions due to its effect on the brain and its effect on someone's daily life. It is important to recognise the presence of a mental health problem and treat it appropriately. Depression and anxiety can (and often do) affect our ability to think and concentrate, they will disrupt our sleep and eating and can therefore perpetuate the symptoms suffered after a head injury.

In this case, it was important for Mary to understand that her persistent symptoms were due to an exacerbation of her underlying mental health condition rather than injury to the brain. If we suffer ongoing symptoms after a head injury it is easy to attribute these to the injury itself rather than exploring whether there may be another cause. The initial injury, symptoms suffered, and social isolation experienced by being off work and not socialising are potent triggers for exacerbating an underlying mental health problem. Therefore, even when the brain has recovered, symptoms due to the mental health problem can continue, leading to a prolongation of symptoms. Recognition of the underling mental health problem and prompt treatment with psychological therapies and possibly medication is therefore important to manage the mental health problems and improve symptoms as seen in this case.

3. Post-traumatic stress symptoms

Understandably, situations that result in a traumatic injury to the head are often the result of a psychologically traumatising event, such as an assault or a road traffic accident. It is therefore common and a **normal** reaction for people to experience post-traumatic stress symptoms following a head injury. These symptoms usually resolve on their own within a few weeks but for some they can persist and become very distressing.

The severity of the head injury itself is often unrelated to how traumatizing the event is from a psychological point of view. Because a milder brain injury results in a briefer period of loss of consciousness and greater memory of the event and its aftermath it is not uncommon for people to experience significant post-traumatic stress symptoms after a mild head injury. *However*, not remembering the event does not necessarily protect you from developing post-traumatic stress symptoms.

Following any traumatising event, it is normal to experience psychological distress that can manifest as physical symptoms including sweating, fast heart rate and rapid breathing. It is important to recognise that this is a **normal** response as the brain processes the event and, in most situations, it resolves over the first few weeks. Equally it is important not to ignore or deny the existence of these symptoms and if they are becoming problematic it is essential to seek help and support.

Post-traumatic symptoms can present in several ways that often co-exist. Common symptoms include re-living the event in nightmares or flashbacks during the day. People often find they are anxious and 'jumpy' as the body adopts a state of heightened alert. This frequently disrupts sleep, impacts on normal brain functioning and leads to increased anxiety. Due to the frightening memories, people suffering post-traumatic stress symptoms will often avoid people and places that remind them of the trauma and prefer not to talk about it.

It can be difficult to know whether we are suffering post-traumatic stress symptoms with all the problems that can occur after a traumatic injury. Following the simple algorithm below can be helpful to know when we should seek help or when to consider whether a friend or family member may be suffering from post-traumatic stress:

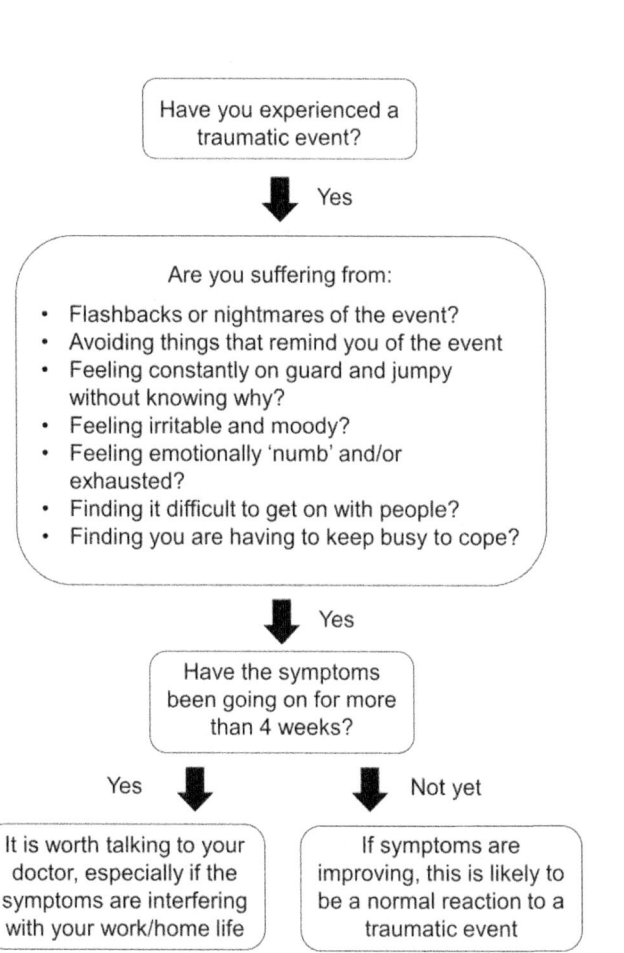

```
Have you experienced a traumatic event?
            ↓ Yes
Are you suffering from:
• Flashbacks or nightmares of the event?
• Avoiding things that remind you of the event
• Feeling constantly on guard and jumpy without knowing why?
• Feeling irritable and moody?
• Feeling emotionally 'numb' and/or exhausted?
• Finding it difficult to get on with people?
• Finding you are having to keep busy to cope?
            ↓ Yes
Have the symptoms been going on for more than 4 weeks?
   ↙ Yes                    ↘ Not yet
It is worth talking to your    If symptoms are
doctor, especially if the      improving, this is likely to
symptoms are interfering       be a normal reaction to a
with your work/home life       traumatic event
```

If you think you are suffering from post-traumatic stress symptoms, there are a few things that you can do in addition to seeing your doctor and getting professional help:

- Try to get back to your normal life, including work and social activities. Although it often feels like the best thing, hiding away, avoiding people, and ruminating on your thoughts is often unhelpful.

- Talk to someone you trust about the event. It is healthy to talk through your feelings and worries in this way and, conversely, trying to tackle something like this on your own can be very difficult. When struggling with these kinds of symptoms it can be hard to see light at the end of the tunnel and another person can prove immensely helpful in making you recognise the need for further support and perhaps assisting you to access it.

- Make sure you eat healthily and exercise regularly. Relaxation exercises including meditation can also be helpful. There are plenty of free Apps and online resources that can help with this.

- It is important to remember that it is **normal** to develop these feelings after a traumatic event. These feelings usually settle on their own with time and you should not feel like a failure or weak because you have developed these feelings. Sometimes these feelings can last longer than you might expect, this does not mean that you will have them for the rest of your life and it is important to remain positive.

- It can often be helpful to go back to where the event happened. Go with someone you trust but do not worry if you cannot face it straight away.

- Alcohol, smoking and other drugs are unhelpful and can make things worse. The initial 'numbing' effects of these substances might feel beneficial but they prevent longer-term recovery. Speak to your doctor and ask for psychological help if you are feeling like the symptoms are getting worse or you are concerned about how long they are lasting.

- When our mind is pre-occupied by other things (such as processing a traumatic event) we can be easily distracted and our concentration is impaired. Try to be mindful of this if doing anything that requires a degree of concentration such as driving, as accidents are more common during this period.

If symptoms persist or cause problems in everyday life, it is important to see your doctor, as there are treatments that can help.

There are numerous psychotherapies or "talking therapies" that can improve symptoms. These tend to focus on helping the brain to process the event and to manage the feelings of fear and distress that it creates. There is one therapy that appears to be quite effective in this situation. It is called Eye Movement Desensitisation and Reprocessing (EMDR). The therapist uses your own eye movements to help the brain to process the flashbacks and your feelings about the event.

Antidepressant medications can also be used and will also help to treat any co-existing depression or generalised anxiety. Medications will often aid the psychotherapies but need to be taken for several months at least and should not be thought of as a magic pill that will instantly fix any psychological issues.

Case study:

Mark was knocked off his bike by a van. He suffered a nasty arm and rib fractures. He had clear memories of the van hitting him and was not knocked unconscious. He had no obvious head injury and was discharged from hospital after an operation on his arm. He was seen in the head injury clinic several weeks later as he reported difficulties with concentrating and thinking. He had been unable to go back to work due to his symptoms and was really worried that he had suffered a significant brain injury that was missed when he came into hospital as the focus was on his arm.

> On further questioning he reported feeling "on edge" and "jumpy" all the time. He was sleeping poorly and experiencing nightmares and flashbacks about the accident. He did not want to leave the house and had been unable to go back to work.
>
> We discussed that the symptoms were suggestive of post-traumatic stress and that this was likely to be causing his other complaints.
>
> We discussed basic measures he could adopt, he was referred to a clinical psychologist with expertise in post-traumatic stress disorder and received EMDR therapy. After a few months symptoms settled and he was able to follow a graded return to work plan.

This case highlights the difficulty we can have in recognising the presence of post-traumatic stress symptoms in ourselves. It can also be difficult for friends, family and even healthcare professionals to identify its presence unless specifically thought about. It is easy to blame persistent symptoms on damage to the brain but identifying the presence of post-traumatic stress is key to understanding the true cause of the symptoms, thereby enabling appropriate therapy and aiding recovery.

It is equally important to recognise that psychological distress can cause many other symptoms including difficulty thinking, headaches and impaired sleep. Managing the psychological aspects is therefore paramount for treating these other symptoms.

4. Difficulties with memory, concentration and speed of thinking

Difficulties with concentration, memory and slowed speed of thinking are common in the initial period after a mild head injury. The brain does a huge amount of work, much of which we take for granted. Not only does it manage our conscious bodily functions like walking, speaking and moving, but it also manages unconscious processes including our breathing, digestion and heartbeat. On top of this, it processes sensory information including vision, hearing and touch whilst also controlling our thinking, emotions and behaviours. It is therefore no surprise that in the recovery period many brain processes that we normally take for granted become more effortful and may not function as well as we would expect.

Even a simple process such as holding a conversation requires multiple different brain functions including hearing the sounds, working out what they mean, thinking of a response and then coordinating the body parts required to generate a reply. These functions happen in different parts of the brain with messages zipping between these regions so fast that the whole process occurs within a fraction of a second. Normally we take this highly complex process for granted. However, if the brain has been injured and needs to recover, it finds these processes harder. Simple conversations suddenly require mental effort; the brain tires quicker and makes errors such as losing concentration and becoming easily distracted. This is normal and is a consequence of the brain recovering. As an analogy, we would not be surprised if we found walking difficult and uncomfortable if we sprained our ankle, and we certainly would not be surprised that we could not run as fast in this situation.

After a mild head injury, it is very rare that these problems with thinking are permanent or due to long-lasting damage to brain structures. They normally resolve over a few weeks to months, but some people do experience problems with memory, concentration or speed of thinking for a longer period than this.

There are several different reasons why people may experience persistent problems with their memory and thinking after a mild head injury that are **not** the result of damage to the brain. These reasons are sometimes referred to under the collective term of a "functional cognitive disorder". Functional cognitive disorder is a common but under-recognised cause of memory or concentration problems. For example, roughly a quarter of patients reporting memory difficulties and seen in memory clinics are diagnosed with a functional cognitive disorder rather than dementia.

The symptoms of a functional cognitive disorder can appear similar to dementia, i.e. misplacing things, forgetting words or losing track of conversations, but they are **not** caused by damage to the brain, instead they are due to the brain not working or functioning as well as we would normally expect. Because they are not due to a structural, visible injury to the brain, it can be hard to understand what is happening. However, it is important to realise that these symptoms are real and not "all in the mind"; an impairment in the brain's functioning is equally as valid as a structural injury to the brain.

Functional cognitive symptoms can happen for a variety of reasons, and often there may be more than one reason. They can develop out of nowhere, but mild head injuries and traumatic events are recognised as common triggers for their development. The table below shows some of the common reasons for a functional cognitive disorder and I will go on to describe them in more detail:

Factors that can impair memory, concentration and thinking

Physical Factors	• Pain • Sleep disturbance • Headaches • Vertigo
Psychological Factors	• Anxiety • Depression • Post-traumatic stress symptoms
Medications and drugs	• Particularly opiate-based but many medications can impair brain function • Alcohol
Over-interpretation of normal brain abilities	

The presence of other physical or psychological problems can impact on our brain's ability to function and are a common cause of functional cognitive symptoms. A useful analogy is a computer. If a computer has multiple 'applications' running or 'windows' open, it will become slow and inefficient as its processing power is being stretched to the limit. At the extreme, the computer may crash and fail to function as we would expect. Likewise, if the brain must deal with other, unrelenting issues including pain or anxiety it will become slow and inefficient. The brain only has so much 'processing power' and, if excessive demands are placed on it, it will have less capacity to carry out its normal functions. This can manifest as an inability to concentrate or to remember everything as we would normally expect. Therefore, it is not that our brain's memory functions are damaged, but that it does not have the capacity to perform these functions to the levels we would normally expect.

Many medications will also affect normal brain functioning. Pain medications (especially opiate-based medications such as codeine) in particular are well-recognised to affect the brain and are a common cause of impaired concentration and brain "fog" after a traumatic injury. These medications are frequently used following trauma, especially if there are multiple injuries. While it is important that pain is treated effectively and that these medications should not be avoided if indicated for pain relief, it is also important to recognise that they can affect brain functions adversely. The message is to stop taking these medications as soon as possible and to understand while taking them that 'thinking problems' may be related to their use rather than because of injury to the brain. Impaired sleep is another common cause of disrupted memory and concentration. Minor head injuries frequently disrupt normal sleep patterns and sleep is fundamental for brain health. If sleep is disturbed, normal brain functions will be impaired, and it is important to optimise sleep and all other aspects of a healthy life if you feel your memory/concentration is not as good as you would expect.

As we mentioned earlier, impaired brain functioning is common in the initial period after a minor head injury due to physical and chemical disturbances within the brain. This initial impairment resolves within a month and usually within a week for nearly all people after a minor injury. However, we sometimes see a persistence of reported problems with memory and/or concentration beyond this time that cannot be attributed to the presence of other physical or psychological factors as discussed above. The reason for the persistence of symptoms in this context is often due to an individual's expectations, their personality type, and their understanding of what happens to the brain after an injury.

To understand how our personality type and beliefs about the head injury and our brain's recovery can affect our perception of our memory it is helpful to describe a scenario that commonly occurs after a minor head injury:

Within the first few days of a minor head injury:

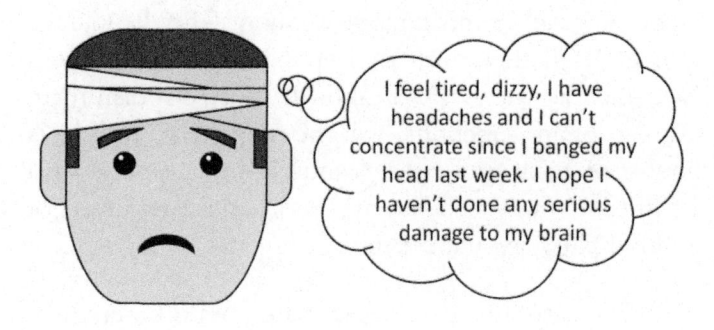

I feel tired, dizzy, I have headaches and I can't concentrate since I banged my head last week. I hope I haven't done any serious damage to my brain

These are normal symptoms and it is normal to have concerns that you may have injured your brain. We often expect to be back to normal within a day or so and if symptoms drag on we can quickly become concerned that there is a serious problem:

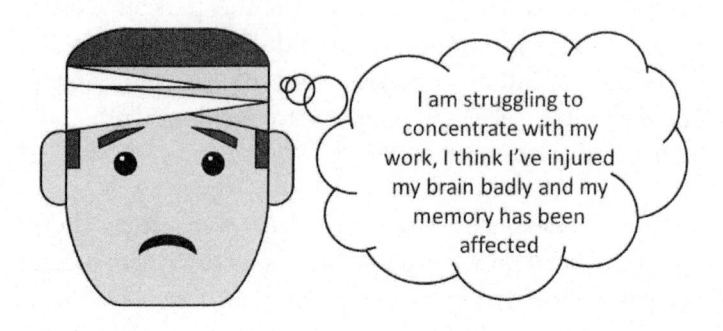

I am struggling to concentrate with my work, I think I've injured my brain badly and my memory has been affected

If the brain is not up and running as fast as we expect, it is easy to start thinking that there has been a significant injury to the brain and that any memory and concentration problems will be permanent. This can lead to our putting pressure on our memory, for example: my memory is bad; I will never remember this person's name. This pressure causes stress, which in turn impairs our memory and we indeed struggle to remember the person's name. In turn this reinforces concerns that our memory has been affected by the head injury and so the vicious cycle continues.

In addition to placing extra pressure on our memory, it is also common to have unrealistic expectations of what our memory was like *before* the accident. We generally consider our memory to be good, but many studies have shown how fallible human memory is. It is common in everyday life to walk into a room and wonder why you went in there or to forget where you put the car keys. These are **normal** attentional lapses that happen to all of us every day. Ordinarily we think nothing of it, brush it off as one of those things and carry on. However, if we are concerned that we have a memory problem or are worried that the recent bang to our head has damaged our brain, we pay more attention to these errors and it is easy to start thinking we have a significant memory problem as we take note of all the times our memory fails us. In summary, it is easy to see how we can develop concerns about our memory (even when it is normal) by becoming more aware of memory failings that all of us suffer every day and are **not** the sign of a memory problem.

Treatment:

The most important aspect of dealing with memory or thinking problems after a minor head injury is to understand the likely recovery and that these problems are **very rarely** due to structural damage to the brain. It is important to recognise that the brain will not be firing on all cylinders for the first few days to weeks after even a minor bang on the head, just as a sprained ankle will be sore to walk on for a similar period of time. Do not become despondent and do not put too much pressure on yourself early on; instead, let the brain recover.

The natural history of this condition is for full brain recovery and for your concentration and memory to improve. However, if symptoms are persisting, consider whether there are other ongoing issues that could be contributing to this, for example, impaired sleep, pain, anxiety, depression or medications that can affect the brain. If these factors are present, then treat them first.

If other psychological and/or physical problems have been addressed and symptoms persist it is a good idea to see your doctor. A detailed assessment of your memory may be helpful in determining whether there are genuine issues or whether you have placed too much expectation on your memory and it is working just fine.

It is useful to keep in mind that memory lapses are common and happen to all of us. Difficulty finding a word, forgetting why we went into a room, and having a memory gap when we have been on 'autopilot' are all very common occurrences in normal, healthy people. It is important not to panic that these lapses are the sign of an underlying brain injury as increasing our focus on our memory has the adverse effect of worsening these symptoms as described above. It is therefore helpful to change how we think about these lapses. For example, when we forget someone's name or have difficulty retrieving a word, remember that this is a normal phenomenon and do not worry that it is the sign of a significant underlying problem.

"Brain-training" may also help as "exercising" our brain's mental abilities can improve confidence in mental abilities and help to rehabilitate the brain after an injury; see the section towards the end of the book that discusses this further.

Case study:

Sarah fell and hit her head on a kitchen cabinet. She was not knocked unconscious but was dazed for several minutes afterwards. She attended A&E, had a normal scan of her head and was discharged with advice. She suffered typical post-traumatic symptoms for a few weeks afterwards and was off work for 2 weeks.

She was seen in the head injury clinic after a couple of months due to reported ongoing difficulties with memory and thinking.

She reported excellent memory prior to the incident and that now she was not as quick with her work, she could jumble up her words and her memory was no longer as good as before.

> She had not had any complaints at work and close friends and family had not said they had noticed any major memory problems.
> She did not report any other physical or psychological symptoms and was not taking any medications regularly. She was fully assessed by a psychologist and her memory was in the upper end of normal.
> We discussed how the initial symptoms and time off work would have led to some deconditioning of her brain but there was almost certainly no long-lasting damage to the brain.. We recommended she undertake some brain training exercises to rehabilitate her memory.

This case highlights how perceptions of having "excellent" memory before an incident can increase the risk of developing subjective memory problems after a head injury. This is not an unusual phenomenon, how many of us look back when we were younger and think "my memory was great then, I guess it gets worse with age". It is true that memory declines with age, but not really until we are in our 60s and beyond. Rather than there being a decline in our memory, this observation of a deterioration is due to a misperception of how good our memory was back then!

It is important to rule out other causative factors and it can be helpful to have an assessment if there are ongoing concerns. However, the acid test is really whether there has been a change in our ability to work, carry out everyday tasks and most importantly whether friends, family and/or work colleagues have noticed a change. If they have not, then it is unlikely that your memory is any different.

In addition, recovering from symptoms and having time off work leads to deconditioning of the brain. It is very common to go back to work after a two-week holiday and to have forgotten your passwords and be slower with your work. Normally, we dismiss this as getting back into work after lounging on a beach for two weeks, but it is easy to see how we may attribute this to an injury to the brain if we have been off work for a few weeks due to a head injury rather than a holiday.

I often recommend that people do puzzles, read or undertake some brain training exercises in this instance as it helps to re-condition the brain – a little bit like prescribing an exercise plan following an arm or leg injury.

5. Dizziness and feeling unsteady

It is very common to feel dizzy and/or unsteady after even a minor head injury. This normally resolves quickly, and most people are back to normal from this point of view within a couple of weeks. However, for some people these feelings persist and can be very disabling and disturbing. Understandably, persistent problems also commonly lead to anxiety and concerns that there may be a significant underlying brain problem. It is quite common therefore to see the development of other symptoms including distress and impairments in concentration, communication and memory in people with persistent feelings of dizziness and imbalance. Correction of the dizziness will often resolve these additional issues.

What causes these feelings of dizziness?

There are many reasons why someone may feel unbalanced, dizzy or light-headed after a head injury and determining the cause is the key to determining correct treatment. We will discuss the common causes and the treatments available but, given the complexity of this issue, if you are suffering persistent symptoms of dizziness, a full medical assessment is likely to be indicated.

The term dizziness means different things to different people and, although this can be difficult, it is important to try to work out exactly what you are experiencing. Generally, when people report feeling dizzy they mean one of the following:

- Feeling light-headed, such as when you stand up quickly or if you are about to faint.

- Feelings of vertigo, this is the sense of the room moving around you or you moving in the room, just like the sensation when you get off a playground roundabout.

- Feelings of being off balance.

- Feelings of 'brain fog' or not being able to think clearly.

Light-headedness

It is common to experience feelings of light-headedness after a minor head injury. This is often due to low blood pressure resulting in insufficient blood getting to the brain. When we stand up or change posture there is a complex system of changes to blood vessels and the heart that maintains our blood pressure and blood flow to the brain. For reasons that are not entirely clear, this system can be disrupted after a head injury. Fortunately, this usually self-resolves within a few weeks and some simple measures to aid resolution include:

- Making sure you are drinking enough fluids.

- Making sure you are exercising (your body will decondition in just a few days if you are inactive)

- Stopping any unnecessary medications (you may need to consult your doctor regarding this)

Important: If you are feeling light-headed or pass out whilst sitting or lying you should get checked out by a health professional to ensure that an alternative cause is not responsible.

Vertigo

Feelings of vertigo can be caused by a disruption to the system that maintains our balance. This system requires the complex integration of signals from different parts of the body which, when collected and computed by the brain, combine to allow us to maintain our balance.

In our inner ear there is a balance apparatus that is sensitive to rotational movement and acceleration. A useful way to think of it can be as the body's 'spirit level'. This is called the vestibular system and is made up of three fluid filled tubes that are oriented in the horizontal, vertical and oblique planes. When the head moves, the movement of the fluid in the tubes generates a signal telling the brain that the head is moving, how fast it is moving and in what direction. In addition, we receive visual input from our eyes and sensory information from our muscles and joints that also tell us if we are moving.

The brain has to integrate all this information and if there is a mismatch or a disruption to this system, we can feel vertiginous, giddy, nauseous and/or disoriented. This is what happens during seasickness, when the signals sent from the inner ear conflict with the visual signals from our eyes. For anyone who has experienced this, it is deeply unpleasant, commonly associated with physical feelings of nausea and often with psychological symptoms including anxiety. However, if given time to readjust, the brain is very good at re-setting the system and accommodating the sensory mismatches. This is what happens when you gain your 'sea-legs' having spent a period of time at sea – your seasickness settles.

Vestibular system
In the inner ear

Visual input

Feedback from muscles and joints

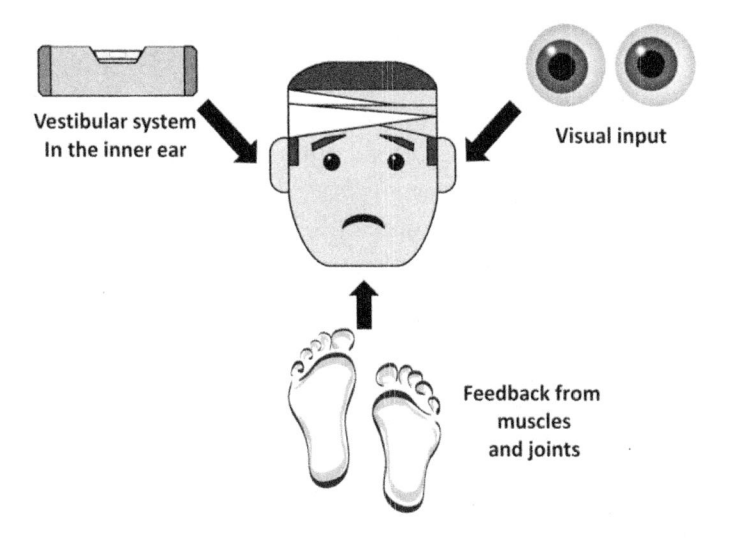

After a minor head injury, vertigo is commonly the result of an inner ear insult or impaired integration of the signals within the brain. Uncommonly, it can be associated with a visual problem although this is usually associated with more obvious symptoms such as double vision. When visual abnormalities are contributing, they are generally easily identifiable by careful clinical examination.

The apparatus in the inner ear can be damaged in several different ways. There may be physical disruption to the inner ear, such as a fracture through the skull in this area. This is usually in the context of a more severe head injury and may be associated with hearing loss. By far the most common cause of disruption to the inner ear after a minor head injury is something called *benign paroxysmal positional vertigo* (or BPPV if this is too much of a mouthful).

BPPV is very common and can occur after even a very minor bang on the head (and commonly occurs outside of the context of head injuries). A crystal in one of the inner ear canals can become dislodged and float freely in the fluid. When the head is turned, this crystal over-stimulates the receptors in the inner ear, sending signals to the brain reporting that the head is turning when it is not. The other inputs, including the eyes, do not report this movement, creating a mismatch in the signals received by the brain from the inner ear and the other organs. This creates the sensation of the room (or your head) spinning rapidly around, like the feeling experienced when you get off a children's roundabout. This feeling usually settles after a few seconds and is commonly caused by a specific movement, such as turning over in bed, looking round or putting your head back. It can be an exceptionally unsettling experience and, although the severe vertigo usually settles within a few seconds to minutes, there can be a prolonged period of feeling slightly off balance afterwards. BPPV usually settles on its own as the crystal finds its way out, but it can be prolonged. In this situation it can lead to many other symptoms including anxiety, impaired balance and disrupted concentration as the person experiencing the BPPV becomes fearful of triggering episodes of vertigo and concerned that it is due to a major underlying brain problem.

BPPV is relatively easy to treat. There are specific manoeuvres that a healthcare professional can do that will clear the crystal from the inner ear canal(s) affected. Therefore, if you are experiencing brief periods of the room spinning on turning your head, seek help and get it treated. It might require further episodes of treatment but often it can be treated in one session. There are also specific exercises that can be done at home called Brandt-Daroff exercises. How to perform these is detailed below, however there are a few words of warning. First, they are not as effective as a trained professional performing similar manoeuvres. Second, make sure you have no neck or back problems that may be exacerbated by these manoeuvres. If you have any neck, back or mobility issues then avoid these exercises and seek professional help. Third, performing these exercises commonly provokes dizziness and it is therefore helpful to have someone else around at last on the first occasion. There is also a small risk that these manoeuvres may worsen symptoms by disrupting other crystals although this is uncommon. Finally, the dizziness may be due to another cause and rather than self-diagnosing and self-treating it is important to have been properly assessed by a healthcare professional to determine the cause of your dizziness. However, if you have been diagnosed with BPPV and have symptoms, these are useful and safe exercises that can be performed at home.

How to do Brandt-Daroff Exercises:

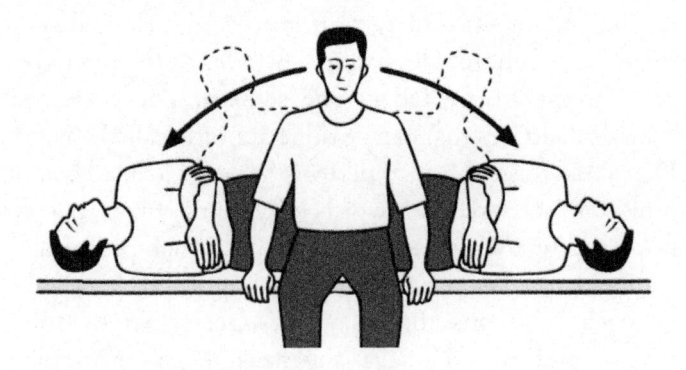

1. Sit upright on the edge of the bed.

2. Turn your head 45 degrees to the left, or as far as is comfortable.

3. Lie down onto your right side and remain in this position for 30 seconds or until any dizziness has subsided.

4. Sit up and turn head back to centre.

5. Turn your head 45 degrees to the right, or as far as is comfortable.

6. Lie down onto your left side and remain in this position for 30 seconds or until any dizziness has subsided.

7. Sit up and turn head back to centre.

The above description is one repetition. The exercises should be performed in a set of 5 repetitions. They should be performed three times a day for two weeks.

A common error in the treatment of vertigo is using anti-sickness medications that suppress the balance apparatus in the inner ear. Given the intense and often disabling nausea, dizziness and imbalance caused by problems with the inner-ear apparatus, medications that suppress these signals and thereby reduce the nausea are often prescribed. Use of these treatments is reasonable for a few days to a week to help alleviate symptoms but longer-term use can prevent the system from rehabilitating itself, thereby prolonging symptoms. Therefore, I normally advise against taking anti-sickness tablets for more than 5 days due to the potential harm it can cause.

Another major cause of vertigo after a head injury is migraine. Vertigo is a relatively common symptom associated with migraines and can occur before, during or after the headache – and sometimes without a headache at all. It can last several minutes to several hours. Treatment of the migraine will also treat the associated vertigo. Migraine is a common cause of intermittent vertigo that persists following a minor head injury in people with ongoing headaches.

There are other, rarer causes of persistent vertigo that require proper assessment by a specialist, but vertigo usually resolves of its own accord and there are effective treatments for many of its causes. The most important points are to treat early to prevent prolongation of symptoms, allow the balance system to rehabilitate and to avoid medications/drugs that worsen symptoms.

Impaired balance

Feeling imbalanced can be separate to dizziness but is again commonly due to a subtle discrepancy in the integration of the signals coming from the inner ear, eyes, muscles and joints.

It is often most noticeable in athletes who suffer a head injury as sports require a high level of balance and coordination. Even a small disruption to this system can become apparent in your ability to perform at your sport. This is of particular importance in this context as impairment in balance can make an athlete more susceptible to injury and is a key motivating factor for making sure symptoms have fully resolved before restarting the sport in question (see the section on Return to contact sports).

In this situation it is important to rehabilitate the body's system of balance. Medications that can impair balance (e.g. opiate painkillers) should be stopped if possible and alcohol consumption reduced or abstained from. Balance exercises, including yoga and Pilates, help to return the system to normal. If we feel imbalanced, our body naturally wants to protect itself by avoiding stressing the balance system. People will often maintain a rigid posture and not move too quickly to prevent feelings of imbalance. However, this will perpetuate the problem as it prevents the balance system from rehabilitating itself.

Case study:

Carol fell backwards whilst ice-skating. She was initially a little dazed and developed a mild headache but otherwise ok. After a couple of days she started to develop dizziness if she turned her head or moved too quickly. She became reluctant to move and was unable to continue her work as a personal trainer as it exacerbated her symptoms.

She was reviewed in the head injury clinic having seen several other doctors who advised her post-concussion symptoms would improve with time. She reported feeling on edge, difficulty concentrating and felt her memory was not as good.

> On examination she had evidence of benign paroxysmal positional vertigo and a corrective procedure was performed. Her symptoms were explained and we discussed how BPPV can generate feelings of anxiety and subjective memory issues.
>
> She required further treatment with a vestibular physiotherapist but symptoms were treated within a few weeks and she was able to resume her personal training job.

This case highlights two important factors. First, some symptoms after a minor head injury do not 'just get better with time'. Instead, they require simple, effective treatments. It is not uncommon for symptoms after a head injury to get attributed to a 'post-concussion syndrome', the implication of which is that time and rest is all that is required to recover. This is often not the correct approach. Benign paroxysmal positional vertigo (BPPV) is a classic example of a cause of vertigo that can be easily treated once diagnosed. Prompt recognition prevents persistent symptoms and avoids unnecessary suffering.

Secondly, BPPV can be associated with a host of other symptoms including anxiety, depression and subjective memory complaints. This may seem odd for a disorder of the inner ear, but the effect caused by the mismatch between signals the brain is expecting and those that it receives can be so profound that other brain processes can go haywire. Treatment of this relatively simple disorder and explanation of the cause of the profoundly disabling symptoms can therefore be all that is required to resolve many persistent symptoms.

6. Light and sound sensitivity

Bright lights, loud noises and strong smells can all be unpleasant after a head injury. This is common in the first few days after a mild head injury. This increased sensitivity to external stimuli is most likely a consequence of the effects of the injury on the brain and its ability to process incoming sensory information. In this early period, the brain is injured and needs to rest. It is therefore understandable that processing a multitude of signals from the eyes, ears and nose upsets the recovering the brain.

As we have discussed, it is reasonable to rest the brain in the early phase and to slowly increase the sensory exposure that the brain must deal with over the first few days to weeks. In contrast, wearing dark glasses or hiding away from light and noise for an excessive period will have the adverse effect of accustoming the brain to darkness and quiet. The brain then adapts to the reduced sensory environment, thereby increasing its sensitivity to normal levels of light and noise. This will hinder the brain's rehabilitation and is the reason why graded increase in sensory exposure is important after the early phase of recovery following a head injury.

If excessive light and noise sensitivity remain for more than the first few weeks, an underlying cause beyond the initial injury should be sought as specific treatment might be required. At this stage it is worth clarifying what is meant by light and noise sensitivity as this will help identify the cause, which is often either due to migraine-type headaches or increased anxiety states:

Migraine-type headaches: The most common cause of persistent light and noise sensitivity after a minor head injury is migraine-type headaches. Sensitivity to light, noise and smells are very common accompaniments of migraine headaches. When light and noise sensitivity is due to migraine, symptoms fluctuate and exposure to light and noise ***exacerbates*** the headache. In addition, light and noise sensitivity due to migraines is often associated with other migrainous features such as nausea, vomiting and brain 'fog'. Treatment of the migraine, as described in the Headache section, will improve the associated light and noise sensitivity.

Anxiety states: A general, constant feeling of being overwhelmed by sensory stimuli can be related to a mental health issue such as anxiety or post-traumatic stress. If we are anxious, our body adopts a state of 'high alert' and our senses are heightened. Normally, our brain filters out most sensory inputs and ignores them, but in a heightened anxiety state this filtering is reduced and the brain can become overwhelmed by all the sensory information it is receiving. This is a useful adaptation for brief periods when we need to be on high alert (for example, our ancestors needed to be able to react quickly and identify potential threats if there was the possibility of attack) but remaining in this state for prolonged periods is detrimental and too many stimuli will overload the brain. Treatment of the underlying mental health issue is the key to managing this feeling of sensory overload.

7. Sleep disturbance and fatigue

Sleep is commonly disrupted after a head injury. There can be many causes for this disruption, and it can exacerbate and/or precipitate many other symptoms – low mood, difficulty concentrating and headaches to name but a few.

There are many ways in which sleep can be disrupted after a head injury. Early on, as the brain is recovering, people often find they are sleeping much more, requiring daytime naps and sleeping longer at night. This is a normal phenomenon and may last a few weeks after a minor head injury. It is a sign that the brain is undergoing repair and needs rest.

However, after this initial period, irregular and unhealthy sleep patterns can develop. Difficulties falling asleep, staying asleep, early morning waking, excessive sleep and disrupted sleep/wake cycles are all common.

There are many causes for disrupted sleep after a brain injury. More severe brain injuries can disrupt the brain structures and chemicals required to control normal sleep behaviours. This is less commonly the case after a minor brain injury and instead it is important to look for and treat other factors that may be contributing to the disrupted sleep.

Anxiety, post-traumatic stress symptoms, and pain are common causes of difficulty falling asleep. Post-traumatic stress can also lead to nightmares that may cause night-time awakenings. There is a complex interplay between mood disturbance (including low mood and anxiety) and sleep problems as one can lead to the other and vice-versa. It can therefore be difficult to differentiate which is causing which, but a pragmatic approach is to manage both the sleep and mental health issues.

It is also easy to develop poor sleep habits. It is common to find that people have continued their daytime naps even when the initial period of recovery is over and they are no longer required. Daytime naps will impair our normal night-time sleep, leading to difficulty falling asleep and maintaining our sleep throughout the night. In addition, if you are not doing as much during the day (maybe due to other issues such as pain or low mood) your night-time sleep will again be disrupted.

Occasionally, a minor head injury can trigger or worsen other sleep problems, for example obstructive sleep apnoea. This is a condition where the walls of the throat relax and narrow during sleep, interrupting normal breathing. This can lead to regularly interrupted sleep, which not only has a big impact on quality of life but also causes many other symptoms such as headache, impaired concentration and sleepiness. Often an individual will snore, have periods where they stop breathing at night and will feel tired during the day. If this is the case, you will need to see your doctor for a comprehensive medical assessment; obstructive sleep apnoea requires prompt and specific treatment.

Fatigue is technically slightly different to tiredness. Sleep and rest will relieve tiredness whereas they do not relieve fatigue. Fatigue is common in all long-term brain conditions. If the brain is working inefficiently for whatever reason, it requires more effort and energy to perform its everyday tasks, resulting in fatigue. Fatigue is very common after a major head injury due to the structural damage to the brain. However, the damage caused by a minor head injury usually resolves and if there is persistent fatigue it is again important to look for other causes such as low mood, chronic pain or anxiety.

Treatments:

When treating abnormalities of sleep after a head injury it is important to identify precisely what the issue is. Is it sleeping too much? Is it difficulty falling asleep or maintaining sleep? Or is it a disrupted sleep-wake cycle? By characterising the specific issue, it is easier to determine the cause and to provide the correct treatment. For example, if there is a problem with falling asleep due to thoughts rushing through your head and heightened anxiety, then these issues should be managed via psychological techniques or anti-anxiety medications rather than prescribing a sleeping tablet, as this will not fix the problem.

After a head injury the brain's ability to adopt a sleeping state can be impaired. Prior to the injury you may have been lucky enough to be able to fall asleep in any kind of environment or after drinking several cups of coffee, but after a head injury it is important to optimise your sleeping environment and sleep-related behaviours as you may now find you are no longer able to sleep as well as before. This is often referred to as "sleep hygiene" and listed below are the measures you can take to try to improve your sleep:

- **Try to establish a bedtime routine**, such as having a bath or reading for a few minutes before going to bed. A light snack or warm milk can also help us to fall asleep.

- **Establish regular sleep times**. This is most useful for the 'getting up time', as you will find it hard to fall asleep if not tired. If you have found that you are getting up later and later, maybe even to late morning or midday, slowly bring it back by setting your alarm clock an hour earlier every few days until you get to the time you want.

- **Avoid napping during the day** as this will impair night-time sleep.

- **Avoid alcohol and caffeine** in the evening and late afternoon as both will impair normal sleep. Alcohol can make us sleepy, but it disrupts the actual sleep we experience and makes it less efficient. Remember that many drinks and foods contain caffeine including chocolate and certain soft drinks – not just tea and coffee.

- **Exercise** is a good way of boosting energy during the day and tiring the body ready for a good night's sleep. However, avoid exercising near to bedtime as this may make it harder to fall asleep.

- **Optimise your bedroom as a place of sleep**:
    - Block out as much light and noise as possible.
    - Ensure that your bed is comfortable and that you are not too hot or too cold.
    - Make your bedroom a place for sleep and do not use it for work.
    - Do not watch television when in bed and limit your exposure to 'screens' for an hour or two before going to sleep.
    - Turn off your phone

- **Try relaxation techniques** before bed including meditation and mindfulness

- **Avoid replaying thoughts over in your head.** If you find you are worrying about things when in bed or thinking about things you need to do, write them down so that you can put them out of your mind and deal with them the following day.

If you have difficulty falling asleep or if you wake up in the middle of the night and then struggle to fall back to sleep, do not panic or worry. Go into another room, have a light snack, wait for 15 minutes or so and then try to go back to sleep.

If these basic measures do not work, then there are several Apps available that can help with sleep. Most adopt a cognitive behavioural approach to improving sleep; this is a process whereby we manage our problems by changing the way we think and behave. These methods can be very effective at managing sleep problems.

It is also worth seeking advice from your doctor as they may be able to refer you to a local insomnia service. They may also consider a short course of sleeping tablets as this can help break the cycle of disrupted sleep. However, it is important to remember that using sleeping tablets for a prolonged period is often unhelpful as they can prevent the resumption of a normal sleep pattern and our brain's ability to fall asleep on its own.

If fatigue is a problem it is important to look for other causative factors including pain, anxiety and depression. It can be helpful to adopt a 'pacing' strategy where you plan your daily activities so that you are not doing too much too soon. The amount you do can be gradually increased to get the body back to functioning at your normal, pre-injury level. There is also some evidence that light therapy, which involves sitting in front of a very bright light for around 45 minutes a day, can help with fatigue levels. Again, if fatigue is a persistent problem see your doctor as they will want to rule out other causes and can help you manage the symptoms.

Case study:

John was assaulted and punched in the face. He briefly lost consciousness and was in hospital for 2 days. He had typical post head injury symptoms for 10 days and was sleeping 12 to 14 hours a day.

He was seen in the head injury clinic 3 months after the injury. He felt tired all the time, he was sleeping until midday and struggled to fall asleep. He had not worked since and his life was severely disrupted.

On closer questioning he was napping during the day and not going to bed until the early hours of the morning. He reported anxiety symptoms related to the assault that kept him awake.

> He was counselled with regards to optimising his sleep hygiene, he was recommended to avoid daytime naps and to set his morning alarm clock an hour earlier every 3 days until he was getting up at 8am. He was encouraged to begin exercise and he was referred for cognitive behavioural therapy for the anxiety symptoms.
>
> Within a few weeks his sleep pattern had normalised, his energy levels increased and his anxiety symptoms were greatly improved. Within a month he was back working.

It is common to develop disrupted sleep patterns and to adopt bad sleep habits after a head injury. A head injury can frequently affect sleep in the early period but once the physical injuries have improved, the poor sleep habits can persist. This can lead to and perpetuate a multitude of other symptoms including mood disturbance and headaches. Commonly, the impaired sleep is felt to be a consequence of the head injury itself but often it is the poor sleep habits themselves that are perpetuating the symptoms.

Adopting good sleep hygiene practices is key to improving symptoms. Often, we find that other symptoms, including mood disturbance, recover as sleep improves. However, identifying whether an abnormal sleep pattern is causing these other symptoms or vice versa is not always easy or even possible – the multiple symptoms are often intimately intertwined, and it is important to address all of them together.

8. Irritability and other changes in personality

Irritability, frustration, feeling low and rapid mood swings are all extremely common after any injury. This is as much due to a combination of the impact of the injury on our normal daily life (e.g. not being able to go to work, exercise or socialise) as well as the physical and psychological effects of the injury itself.

After even a mild head injury, it is common for people to experience a disruption to their normal work and social lives for a period of time. This is especially true if there are other injuries besides the head injury that affect our ability to take part in normal daily life. This can be very frustrating and will manifest regularly as a change in behaviour and/or personality. As things recover and normal life resumes these issues tend to improve.

In addition, persistent physical symptoms such as headache, dizziness or disrupted sleep will impact on mood and behaviour. Most of us at some point in our lives will have suffered a period of disrupted sleep or prolonged pain and are only too aware of how that made us grumpy and irritable. It is the same after a head injury, which is commonly responsible for transient changes in both mood and behaviour.

It is also important to monitor for the presence of mental health problems, as anxiety, post-traumatic stress symptoms and depression can all manifest as changes in behaviour and personality.

It is therefore imperative to address any ongoing physical symptoms (e.g. impaired sleep or pain) as well as any mental health issues and to treat these appropriately. In addition to these simple measures, psychological or "talking" therapies can be helpful with managing changes in mood or behaviour and occasionally medications including anti-depressants are also used.

It is important to remember that these changes are some of the most common issues we see in the clinic and are normally the consequence of the other factors discussed above. However, if changes in personality or behaviour are becoming problematic seek help from your doctor, as they will be able to address any causative factors and help direct treatment.

9. Problems with vision

"Blurred vision" is a typical symptom described after a minor head injury. It is usually short-lived and settles within a few days. If vision problems persist beyond a few days or the symptoms are more severe than slight blurring, then it is advisable to have your eyes properly assessed by an optician or eye doctor.

The symptom of "blurred vision" commonly experienced and reported by people early after a minor head injury is likely to be a consequence of minor disruption to the vision processing pathways in the brain and/or the control of eye movements.

The vision system is incredibly complex and finely tuned. Have you ever thought how impressive it is that we can move both our eyes in perfect unison even when following a fast-moving object? The slightest discrepancy in movement between our two eyes will result in each eye transmitting a slightly different image to the brain. This will result in double vision that will appear blurry as the two separate images from each eye will not overlap exactly:

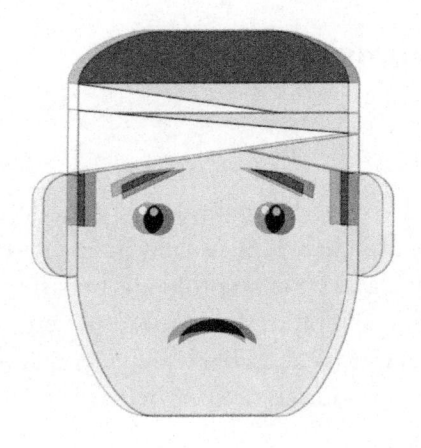

The brain is responsible for controlling this coordinated movement of our eyes. Therefore, just as with many other brain processes following a head injury, if this system is not working perfectly our vision will appear blurred. This usually resolves very quickly but if the double vision persists or is particularly noticeable on looking in a certain direction you should be assessed by an eye doctor, as sometimes there can be more significant damage to the visual system that may require special treatment.

In addition to controlling our eye movements, the brain is responsible for processing the visual information our eyes receive. This too is a highly complex process, with cells at the back of the eyeball (the retina) converting the light signals they receive into electrical signals. These electrical signals are transmitted via nerve cells through to the back of the brain to an area called the occipital cortex where they are processed with further onward projections throughout the brain to allow us to create a visual image of the world around us. Again, it is easy to imagine that if the brain is not working at full capacity and is recovering from an injury, this complex process will become more effortful and we may feel that our vision is not as good as it was before. As the brain recovers, this too will improve and, ordinarily, vision returns to normal very quickly.

If the vision problem is only present in one eye then this may be due to damage to that eye; for example, the front of the eye can be scratched during trauma or the retina at the back of the eyeball can be damaged or torn. Any visual problem that is isolated to just one eye should be assessed immediately by an eye specialist.

Intermittent visual symptoms after a head injury are often due to migraine-type headaches. As discussed earlier, headaches after even a minor head injury are common and most resemble a migraine-type headache. Migraines are not *just* a headache but are a brain disorder with many associated features including visual disturbance. The classic visual disturbance associated with migraines is jagged lines or kaleidoscopic vision. However, migraine can also present with blurring, sparkly lights or distorted vision. The important point is that these visual disturbances are **intermittent**, usually change over time and last seconds to minutes. It is also important to note that, although a headache often follows these visual changes, this is not always the case.

Certain medications that are commonly prescribed following a head injury (including some pain medications and anti-depressants) can cause dry, gritty eyes that may give the impression of blurred or affected vision. Simple eye drops or switching/stopping the causative medications is likely to help but discuss this with your doctor first.

Finally, it is not uncommon for a head injury to unmask an underlying issue that was present before the injury but may not have been particularly noticeable. Head injuries can exacerbate a refractive error (i.e. long or short-sightedness) that requires glasses or even an underlying cataract. Therefore, if symptoms of blurry vision persist, see your optician to see whether there is another cause that can be remedied.

10. Hearing problems

A variety of hearing problems are common after minor head injuries. Tinnitus (hearing a sound, often a ringing or buzzing, when there is no external sound source) and sensitivity to noises are the most common. Like most post-traumatic symptoms, these often improve within a few days to weeks. If they do not or are associated with other features such as hearing loss or vertigo (a feeling that the room is spinning), then they should be assessed by a doctor as there may be a treatable underlying cause.

Tinnitus is the perception of a noise without the presence of an external noise source. It is often a high-pitched ringing or buzzing sound. It is not uncommon in the general population but is more common after a head injury. There are many different reasons why it may develop after a head injury and these include damage to the ear, the nerves carrying the sound information from the ear to the brain and damage to the brain itself. Normally tinnitus resolves within a few days to weeks and is not due to a worrying cause. However, occasionally it can be due to particular damage that requires investigation and treatment. If tinnitus does not resolve in time with other typical symptoms (e.g. dizziness, tiredness and headache) it is recommended to see your doctor for an assessment. In addition, if the tinnitus is pulsatile (matches your heart-beat) and/or is associated with hearing loss or vertigo, then you should see your doctor – there might be an underlying problem that needs to be addressed.

Although in the majority of cases there is no concerning cause for tinnitus after a minor head injury, it is still an unpleasant symptom that is frequently associated with disrupted sleep, emotional distress, depression and anxiety and can affect concentration, memory and attention. Understanding what is happening and recognising that it is not due to a worrying cause is the first step in treating tinnitus. Talking therapies can also help to address the associated feelings of distress and manage coping with this disabling symptom.

There is also a more specific treatment called sound therapy. Sound therapy or sound enrichment uses the concept of habituation to reduce the impact of the tinnitus. Tinnitus is commonly worse in quiet environments as there is nothing else to distract the brain. Therefore, sound therapy works on the principle of exposing the brain to a constant external sound, with the aim of improving the brain's ability to filter out the internally generated tinnitus. This can be achieved via portable sound generators or wearable ones that look like small hearing aids.

Several medications and herbal remedies have been trialled but the evidence for their effectiveness is limited. It is therefore worth seeking help if tinnitus is causing a problem and as with all symptoms following a head injury, adopting a heathy lifestyle, and treating sleep and mental health problems can all help with the symptoms. Further information and support are available at the

British Tinnitus Association website www.tinnitus.org.uk.

> **Tinnitus features after a mild head injury that warrant a review by a healthcare professional**
>
> - Pulsatile tinnitus
> - Associated with severe vertigo
> - Associated with hearing loss
> - Is causing distress/worry
> - Has not resolved within a few days to weeks with the other typical post head injury symptoms
> - Tinnitus present in just one ear

Noise sensitivity is also common after a head injury. This is normally combined with sensitivity to light and is discussed earlier in Chapter 6. If it is isolated sensitivity to sound then it is important to have this assessed to make sure there is no hearing problem causing this.

Hearing loss is unusual after a minor head injury and warrants review by a hearing specialist to look for damage to the hearing apparatus.

Case study:

Maria was knocked off her bicycle by a car. She was briefly knocked unconscious and injured her shoulder. She developed frequent, severe headaches following the incident, post-traumatic stress symptoms and tinnitus.

She was assessed in the head injury clinic and was diagnosed with a persistent post-traumatic headache with migraine features, post-traumatic stress disorder and persistent tinnitus present in both ears that had a constant, high-pitched quality.

> She was referred for a full hearing assessment that was completely normal, she received treatment for the headaches and medication and psychological therapy for the post-traumatic stress symptoms.
>
> She was reassured there were no worrying findings from the hearing assessment and she was referred for sound therapy and psychological therapy but she declined. The headaches and post-traumatic stress symptoms improved over several months and at the same time the tinnitus resolved.

If specifically asked about, a significant proportion of people report tinnitus after a minor head injury. It is important to rule out an injury to the hearing apparatus and to identify and treat other issues such as the headache and post-traumatic stress disorder as in this case.

There is a complex relationship between headaches, particularly migraine, and tinnitus, with tinnitus occurring more frequently in people who suffer with migraine. In addition, anxiety is a common side effect of tinnitus and, in turn, is recognised to **worsen** tinnitus. Therefore, treating these other symptoms can be effective at treating the tinnitus but this should be in combination with standard tinnitus treatments.

PART 3:
Specific issues following a concussion

Getting back to work, exercise and education

Getting back to work

The specifics regarding returning to work obviously depend on several factors for each individual, not least the nature of work, the severity of the injury and any persistent symptoms that may be present. For example, intermittent vertigo/dizziness poses a far greater risk for someone who works at heights – the building trade is a classic example – than for someone working in an office environment. However, there are some guiding principles that all people can follow, and it is highly recommended to have early discussions with your workplace's occupational health team and managers.

Graded return:

First, and perhaps most importantly, a graded return to work is vital. Even if you feel completely fine whilst resting at home, it is invariably the case that returning to the stresses and demands of work is harder than people expect. It is not uncommon for this process to exacerbate a headache or other symptoms. I frequently see people who have tried to rush back into work. As a result, they have aggravated their symptoms and have ended up far worse after a few weeks. They then find themselves unable to work for a prolonged period. In contrast, if they had taken their time and adopted a graded return to work, they would have taken less time off in the long run.

The graded return is a very individual process and only you can decide the fine details. Some people need a couple of half days, feel fine and are then able to rapidly increase their workload to normal levels. Others take several weeks to function at their pre-injury level.

In judging the speed of return to employment, it is important to recognise that you need to tread a fine line between doing too much, which will overload the brain and hinder recovery, and doing too little, which will lead to deconditioning and make any level of work feel effortful.

To help judge this I find a useful analogy is going to the gym; if we go to the gym but do not get out of breath then we are not improving our fitness, equally, if we decide to run a marathon having not run further than a few hundred metres we are likely to end up in a heap and unable to run for a long time. Therefore, it is important to stretch yourself to get back to previous levels of functioning at work and to recognise that you are likely to feel more tired initially but to slowly increase work levels rather than going from 0 to 100mph over the course of a few days.

Realistic expectations:

Second, have realistic expectations. If your job requires a high demand on thinking abilities, do not be surprised that you are not up to 100% straight away. Your work colleagues and managers need to appreciate this, and it is often better to start with easier jobs before moving onto more complex ones. You may also require supervision initially, especially if your job involves high risk situations, for example if you are a surgeon or operate potentially dangerous machinery.

Persevere:

Third, do not become despondent if symptoms worsen. This is common and is merely a consequence of the fact you are placing more demands and strain on the brain. This is **not** a sign that you have done permanent damage to the brain.

If we use the analogy of a sprained ankle, we would not be surprised if when we started running again the ankle was sore and running was more effortful than before. We would probably expect that even if the ankle were pain free at rest, it may hurt slightly on running but that this would improve with time and practise. We would also expect to be able to do more vigorous exercise over time as our ankle recovered and we got it used to moving again after a period of inactivity. Equally, most of us realise that not exercising an ankle after an injury will lead to it stiffening and becoming weaker. This is the same with the brain. Resting at home may not produce any symptoms but placing demands on the brain may exacerbate symptoms. It is important to persevere, as avoiding these demands will lead to deconditioning and a slower recovery. Equally, the brain has not been performing all its usual tasks and therefore there is a 'rehabilitation' element required to get the brain back up and running to its usual capacity.

Treat symptoms:

Fourth, make sure that any residual symptoms are being optimally treated. Returning to a work environment is likely to exacerbate any persistent symptoms. Therefore, make sure you have consulted with your doctor if you have ongoing headaches, dizziness or other symptoms.

Preparation:

Finally, it is advisable to prepare as much as you can before starting back at work. Try your usual commute before you intend to start back, going through a busy railway station can be a stressful process with huge amounts of sensory stimuli that can easily exacerbate symptoms. Practice cognitively demanding tasks including reading and using a computer to increase your ability to concentrate. If your job is physically demanding, make sure you can cope with the physical demands required prior to encountering them in a work situation.

Getting back to exercise

Return to exercise should follow a similar pattern. Again, a graded return is key and a recognition that although you may have been running marathons before the head injury, the body rapidly deconditions and it is important to build up and not put too much pressure on yourself or the brain. Migraines in particular can be worsened by exercise and if you are suffering from headaches and you find exercise induces them, taking an anti-inflammatory medication, such as ibuprofen, prior to exercise can be a useful way to prevent the headache. However, this is not a long-term solution and these medications should not be taken on a regular basis due to the risk of medication overuse headaches and irritation to the stomach.

I recommend initiating some form of exercise as soon as possible, even if it is a simple walk. After a mild head injury 24-48 hours should be the maximum amount of complete rest required and gentle exercise is important to prevent deconditioning and prolongation of symptoms.

Getting back to education

Returning to school or higher education can be slightly more complicated. There is often the added pressure of an imminent exam or the concern of falling behind if too much time is missed. These are understandable concerns, but the same process of a graded return should be adopted; all too frequently we see school children rush back into schoolwork in an attempt not to fall behind only to find that they subsequently need to take more time off school later on.

Schools and Universities are much better informed regarding the consequences of head injuries than they used to be, and it makes sense to have early conversations and make a plan. We are all different and it maybe that a week of half days is plenty for some to get back up to speed, but for others a more drawn-out process may be required.

The brain has a limited capacity in how much it can do. After an injury, this capacity is reduced while recovery happens. Therefore, it is sensible to focus on the most important factors first, for instance attending key classes initially and leaving extracurricular activities until schoolwork can be fully completed. More rest and sleep are also likely to be needed. Avoiding diversions and distractions can also be helpful in the recovery stage. For example, eating a packed lunch in a quiet area rather than in a busy canteen will produce fewer distractions and will help to conserve mental energy as the brain has fewer sensory inputs to filter and process.

Return to contact sports

The recognition, understanding and management of head injuries in sport have improved greatly over the last few years. Most sports have developed guidelines surrounding the recognition of a head injury, its management and return-to-play protocols. It is worth accessing the specific guidance from your sport's governing body (most have detailed guidelines) as there may be some sport-dependent differences.

From a general point of view, it is worth understanding the aim of sporting head injury guidelines and the aspects they do not necessarily cover.

Most sports have published guidelines and education regarding the recognition of head injuries, the need for removal from play and how to restart playing. It is recognised that the risk of a further injury (to the head or any other part of the body) is greatly increased after a head injury. This is presumably due to the effect a head injury has on our balance, coordination and judgement that makes us vulnerable to a further injury. **Therefore, it is important to identify if you or someone else has had a potential head injury and remove yourself or them from the game to prevent a further injury.**

It should be noted that individuals suffering a head injury are often unable to make the judgement about whether they have had a head injury and about the need to stop playing. It is therefore important to adopt a cautious approach, if there is any doubt about whether someone has suffered a head injury, remove them from the game and assess them.

We talked earlier about second-impact syndrome. There is some debate as to whether this is a rare event that occurs after a second head injury that has followed soon after and while recovering from an initial head injury or whether a preceding head injury is irrelevant and it is instead a very rare event that can happen after a single, isolated head injury. **Either way**, given the increased risk of a further injury, if the brain has not recovered from a head injury it is important that someone should be taken off the field of play immediately and should not play again until they have fully recovered.

Most sporting bodies provide guidelines regarding the return-to-play process following a head injury. Some stipulate strictly defined periods of rest from the sport in question and most provide guidance on a stepwise process of return to play. As a general principle, most guidelines recommend starting with simple exercise and increasing in intensity only when symptom-free at each stage. For example, start initially with light aerobic activity such as a gentle jog. If this can be completed without symptoms then progress to more specific sport-related activities such as sprints or changing direction, this can then increase to non-contact training drills, followed by full contact practice and finally return to play. If there are symptoms at any stage, then the player should return to the previous level, treat any ongoing issues (e.g. headache, sleep issues or too many medications) before slowly increasing the intensity of training again.

Governing bodies for contact sports have also recognised the need to reduce the risk and severity of head injuries. Most are taking steps to make their sport safer, but most forms of physical exercise are likely to involve some risk of injuring the head. It is important to recognise that exercise and team sports provide many benefits in terms of physical and mental health and these positives should not be forgotten when we consider the potential risks of any sport.

Persistent symptoms after a sporting head injury:

What happens if symptoms do not improve after a period of rest and appropriate graded return to activity? Just as with any minor head injury, there are a proportion of individuals who will develop persistent symptoms after a sports-related head injury. As discussed in the context of non-sports related head injuries, there are multiple reasons why this might be and the chances of it being due to permanent brain damage are unlikely. Again, it is worth re-iterating that the development of persistent symptoms after a head injury is a **separate** issue to the risk of developing a progressive dementia like chronic traumatic encephalopathy many years later. Instead, seeking expert help is recommended to help determine the cause of the persistent symptoms and treating appropriately. In addition, a more prolonged period of rest from the sport in question is likely to allow full recovery.

For those who have suffered more than one minor head injury, it is important to assess why this might be happening. Is there something in the way they are playing the sport in question that is exposing them to a greater risk of suffering a head injury or do they seem more prone to suffering a head injury? In this situation, a longer rest period is likely to be required and careful thought about minimising future risk and continuing with the sport are needed.

Risk of future dementia:

As discussed earlier, there is now good evidence supporting a link between repeated minor head injuries and progressive forms of dementia, specifically chronic traumatic encephalopathy. As discussed in more detail above, there is still a lot that is unknown about this association. In particular, how many head injuries are required and how severe do they have to be? Certain individuals are also probably more predisposed either due to genetic or lifestyle factors. Again, it is important to remember that physical sports provide many benefits, and these positives should not be forgotten. It is not possible for anyone to be able to give clear guidance on the risk as there is so much we still do not know about this area. However, minimising the exposure to head injuries and recovering fully from any head injury sustained are sensible and important considerations.

However, for people who continue to have head injuries or persistent post-head injury symptoms a consideration of whether to continue playing the sport in question needs to be made. Everyone is unique and everyone will have different priorities when it comes to making a decision such as this. However, for all individuals a balanced approach to weighing up the pros and cons is important when deciding whether to continue. One must consider how important playing the particular sport is to them. There is clearly a difference between someone who plays for fun and someone who is paid to play the sport as a professional. Second, the potential risk of developing a future neurodegenerative condition needs to be considered and the potential risk of causing permanent neurological injury with repeated head injuries. It is also important to think about the effect of a head injury on your current work or studies, even for people who make a full recovery there is a period when the brain is recovering and therefore people suffering repeated head injuries will impact on other aspects of their lives. Ultimately, this is a decision that only the individual in question can make and unfortunately there is much we do not know about the future risks. Therefore, one must consider the potential for future complications, the current impact of symptoms and the benefits of continuing with the sport.

Diet and supplements

Various diets, foods and supplements have been claimed to aid recovery after a head injury. These claims come with plausible mechanisms of action, for example diets based on foods high in anti-oxidants that calm the inflammation in the brain and/or foods rich in substances that are the core building blocks for brain cells and therefore promote brain repair. These foods also tend to be foods that most would consider to be present in any healthy diet (e.g. fruit, vegetables, fish etc.) and there is no clear evidence that these particular "brain health" diets speed up recovery beyond the fact they constitute a normal healthy diet.

Foods proposed to help brain recovery include those high in antioxidants, such as blueberries, strawberries, kale and dark chocolate. Antioxidants clear up free radicals, these are molecules that can damage cells and are more abundant in the brain following injury. This is a plausible mechanism and foods high in antioxidants are important in a healthy diet, however, there is no evidence that eating hundreds of blueberries a day is any more helpful than making these foods an element of your normal healthy diet.

Omega-3 fatty acids are important structural components of cell membranes, facilitate various brain cell functions and have anti-inflammatory effects. Fatty fish including salmon and mackerel as well as walnuts and soybeans are high in omega-3 fatty acids. There have been studies in animals showing high dose supplements of omega-3 fatty acids promote recovery after a brain injury but there is no good evidence that it helps after a mild head injury in humans. However, whilst taking high dose supplements of Omega-3 may not necessarily speed up recovery, Omega-3 rich foods are recommended in a healthy diet.

Certain specialist diets, including high fat diets and reduced calorie diets, have been proposed as having potential beneficial effects on brain recovery. There is no good evidence for this in the context of recovery from a head injury and they may in fact have a harmful effect.

Overall, despite the fact there is no clear evidence that a particular diet or supplement will speed recovery, it is important to remember that the brain uses 20% of the body's energy. It therefore makes sense that we would want to provide the brain with a good healthy diet to provide this energy whilst it is recovering, and it is likely that the brain will be more susceptible to the effects of a 'bad' diet than pre-injury. We have all experienced the sluggish effects of a large, unhealthy meal and it is highly likely that these effects will be amplified after a head injury. This is also true for alcohol. The effects of alcohol on balance and thinking are more prominent after a head injury and therefore it should be avoided during the recovery period.

A healthy diet includes fruits, vegetables, whole grains, lean meats, and a couple of portions of fatty fish per week. Avoid sugary foods and drinks, foods high in salt, processed and fatty foods. Stay well hydrated by drinking plenty of water and remember 'everything in moderation'

– just because a handful of blueberries is good for you, a bucketful is unlikely to be any better and some foods or supplements in excess may be harmful.

"Brain-Training"

There are numerous 'brain-training' platforms that claim to improve memory, concentration and overall brain 'power'. 'Brain-training' has become a controversial area; it has grown into a multi-billion dollar business but there is ongoing debate about whether it is effective at improving brain function.

Is brain-training effective? There is no simple answer to this. It does appear that doing brain-training exercises improves our ability at that specific brain-training task. For example, if we practice learning a string of numbers, we will get better at reciting a string of numbers. However, the evidence that this translates into improved general brain function is limited. In other words, getting good at remembering a sequence of numbers does not seem to improve our general IQ.

Second, any task requiring concentration and brainpower will improve our brain's abilities. For example, doing crosswords, puzzles, card games or computer games will improve the cognitive functions related to those activities. Computer games improve concentration and reaction times and crosswords can improve verbal skills. Therefore, it is not necessary to pay large amounts of money for specific 'brain-training' programmes as the effects can be gained using other, readily available, free sources.

The most important aspect for aiding recovery is to follow a graded return to full brain activity. We want to avoid the brain deconditioning too much by not doing anything, but we also want to avoid the 'boom and bust' scenario mentioned earlier where we overload the recovering brain before it is ready and worsen symptoms as a result. Therefore, as with physical exercise, after a brief period of rest you should aim to slowly increase the demands you place on your brain. Do not lie in bed for several days doing nothing and then attempt to complete your 4 hours of mathematics homework. Even simple tasks, such as watching a television programme or reading a magazine article require concentration. Therefore, aim to manage these simple tasks first and then gradually build up to more complex tasks so that you are ready to manage the complex demands of work or study.

It is not uncommon for people to feel that they are not back to their normal level of brain functioning after a minor head injury. This can lead to concern that they have irrevocably damaged their brain and they will never be able to perform at the same level as before. This is rarely the case and there are several other more common reasons for this to occur:

First, make sure you have not deconditioned too much. As we mentioned earlier, if you do nothing with your arm it will weaken, stiffen up and the muscles will waste within a matter of days. The brain will also rapidly decondition. Most of us have experienced the post-holiday scenario where we return to studying or work and have found we are much slower and not as confident in our work. We normally brush this concern off, attribute it to lying on a beach for 2 weeks and within a few days we are functioning at our normal levels. Therefore, do not be surprised if you are not functioning at your normal levels for a while if you have taken time to recover from a head injury. Persevere and often it will return. It is also at this stage that training the brain can be helpful. Brain-training exercises can be used or playing puzzles and card times can also be effective.

Second, make sure there are no other persistent symptoms that are impairing your brain function. Common symptoms that will impair our ability to think, concentrate and remember include headaches, sleep disturbance, anxiety and/or depression. If these issues are present, brain training will not help and may even worsen the symptoms. It is important to treat these symptoms to allow the brain to return to normal levels of functioning.

Third, we sometimes over-estimate our previous abilities, the so-called 'rose-tinted spectacles' phenomenon. Even outside of the context of head injuries this will occur, people will often recollect that 10 years ago "I could remember everything". Brain-training can help in this situation as it can improve confidence in our abilities and allows us to realise that, with practise, we can improve our brain's abilities.

Overall, it is important to exercise our brain during recovery. Brain-training in itself is not going to be harmful (unless we overload the brain too early) and probably will help our road to recovery in certain situations, but there are simple, free alternatives that are likely to be as beneficial as dedicated brain-training platforms.

Driving and flying

Most people can return to driving relatively soon after a minor head injury. Exact rules will depend on local driving regulations and these are country specific. Normally, if you have suffered only a minor head injury with no changes on a brain scan and no more than a brief period of loss of consciousness or altered mental status then you are allowed to drive after symptoms stopping you from driving safely have resolved *(please check your National or State specific rules)*. This is only true for normal driving licences; commercial licences for heavy goods vehicles etc. have different and often much stricter regulations and even minor head injuries will more often than not mandate a period of not driving and the relevant driving authority should be informed.

There are several general issues that need to be considered when deciding about driving which we will discuss below. However, if there are any doubts you should discuss with your driving authority and/or healthcare professional as failure to declare a medical condition that has the potential to affect driving will usually invalidate insurance and you can be fined or prosecuted.

Symptoms affecting driving:

As mentioned above, even if you suffered the most minor of head injuries, all symptoms that may affect driving must be fully resolved to allow resumption of driving. You should be able to concentrate for long enough periods, be able to react quickly to unexpected situations and judge distances and speeds of other vehicles and objects. Determining whether you have symptoms that preclude you from driving may involve an element of judgement. For example, if you are suffering intermittent episodes of vertigo on turning your head (e.g. BPPV) is this enough to make you unsafe to drive? I would argue it does and needs to be declared to the driving authority and discussed with your healthcare professional. In addition, excessive tiredness is another common complaint that makes driving dangerous and should be fully resolved.

Driving is a complex task requiring the assimilation of a lot of sensory information. Therefore, even subtle impairments in thinking, speed of information processing and attention are likely to impair your ability to drive. It can be difficult to decide whether we are safe to drive and it is often helpful to ask friends and relatives what they think. It is also possible to undergo a driving evaluation in most countries as ultimately the best way to test your ability to drive is by being assessed doing the task itself. This is the best way to decide and I often recommend it for people who are in doubt.

Other factors:

Even if all symptoms have resolved, it is important to make sure there are no other issues preventing safe driving. In particular, what was the cause of the head injury? If it was due to a fall precipitated by an unexplained loss of consciousness or a seizure, then this in itself is a contraindication to driving. Medications can also affect driving, for example some painkillers can cause drowsiness.

Finally, a head injury can induce an epileptic seizure. Seizures are a common reason why people are not allowed to drive and most authorities stipulate a period of 'seizure freedom' before being allowed to drive again. A seizure in the context of a head injury is slightly different and, in the UK at least, a seizure "occurring at the very moment of impact of a head injury" does not necessarily require driving to cease unless it exposed an underlying predisposition to seizures. A seizure occurring after the actual injury will, however, be subject to the usual rules regarding seizures and driving.

If there is any doubt, I re-iterate, it is safest to discuss with your driving regulator and/or healthcare professional.

Flying:

There are no particular rules regarding flying after a minor head injury. The lower pressure in an aircraft cabin can exacerbate symptoms and travelling between time zones is liable to worsen symptoms, particularly migraine. It is important to be aware of these factors and decide based on the importance of the trip and how you are managing with symptoms. There is no suggestion that flying soon after a minor head injury causes any long-term problems and usual measures to optimise flying well-being should be taken including staying hydrated, avoiding alcohol and regular stretching and moving.

Where to get extra help

Headway: www.headway.org.uk

The United Kingdom Acquired Brain Injury Forum: ukabif.org.uk

NHS Choices: www.nhs.uk/conditions/Concussion/Pages/Introduction.aspx

Brain Line: www.brainline.org

Headinjurysymptoms.org: www.headinjurysymptoms.org

Child Brain Injury Trust: www.childbraininjurytrust.org.uk

The Children's Trust: www.thechildrenstrust.org.uk

Mind: www.mind.org.uk

British Tinnitus Association: www.tinnitus.org.uk

Printed in Great Britain
by Amazon